Interpretation of Pulmonary Function Tests
A Practical Guide

Second Edition

Interpretation of Pulmonary Function Tests
A Practical Guide

Second Edition

Robert E. Hyatt, M.D.

Emeritus Member
Division of Pulmonary and Critical Care Medicine
and Internal Medicine
Mayo Clinic
Emeritus Professor of Medicine and of Physiology
Mayo Medical School
Rochester, Minnesota

Paul D. Scanlon, M.D.

Consultant
Division of Pulmonary and Critical Care Medicine
and Internal Medicine
Mayo Clinic
Professor of Medicine
Mayo Medical School
Rochester, Minnesota

Masao Nakamura, M.D.

Vice-Director
Keihai-Rosai Hospital
Fujihara-machi Sioyagun
Tochigi-ken, Japan

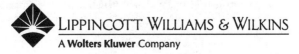

LIPPINCOTT WILLIAMS & WILKINS
A **Wolters Kluwer** Company

Philadelphia • Baltimore • New York • London
Buenos Aires • Hong Kong • Sydney • Tokyo

Acquisitions Editor: Joyce-Rachel John
Developmental Editor: Erin McMullan
Production Editor: Jeff Somers
Manufacturing Manager: Ben Rivera
Cover Designer: Christine Jenny
Compositor: TechBooks
Printer: Maple Press

Published by
LIPPINCOTT WILLIAMS AND WILKINS
530 Walnut Street
Philadelphia, PA 19106 USA
LWW.com

Printed in the United States of America

9 8 7 6 5 4 3 2

Library of Congress Cataloging-in-Publication Data

Hyatt, Robert E.
    Interpretation of pulmonary function tests : a practical guide /
Robert E. Hyatt, Paul D. Scanlon, Masao Nakamura. — 2nd ed.
      p. ; cm.
    Includes bibliographical references and index.
    ISBN 0-7817-3682-X
    1. Pulmonary function tests.   I. Scanlon, Paul D. (Paul David)
II. Nakamura, Masao, M. D.   III. Title.
    [DNLM: 1. Respiratory Function Tests.   2. Lung Diseases—
diagnosis.   WF   141 H992i 2003]
RC734.P84I I93   2003
616.2'4075—dc21   2002043394

Care has been taken to confirm the accuracy of the information presented and to describe generally accepted practices. However, the authors and publisher are not responsible for errors or omissions or for any consequences from application of the information in this book and make no warranty, express or implied, with respect to the currency, completeness, or accuracy of the contents of the publication. Application of this information in a particular situation remains the professional responsibility of the practitioner.

    The authors and publisher have exerted every effort to ensure that drug selection and dosage set forth in this text are in accordance with current recommendations and practice at the time of publication. However, in view of ongoing research, changes in government regulations, and the constant flow of information relating to drug therapy and drug reactions, the reader is urged to check the package insert for each drug for any change in indications and dosage and for added warnings and precautions. This is particularly important when the recommended agent is a new or infrequently employed drug.

    Some drugs and medical devices presented in this publication have U. S. Food and Drug Administration (FDA) clearance for limited use in restricted research settings. It is the responsibility of the health care provider to ascertain the FDA status of each drug or device planned for use in their clinical practice.

Contents

Preface

The first edition of *Interpretation of Pulmonary Function Tests* was well received and met our goal of appealing to a wide, varied audience of health professionals. In the second edition, we added a section to expand our discussion of lung mechanics. We emphasize the mechanical impairments faced by patients with obstructive lung disease and those with pulmonary fibrosis. Three cases were added in which special tests of lung mechanics are informative.

The illustrative cases were very popular in the first edition. We have added cases that demonstrate congestive heart failure mimicking pulmonary fibrosis, the importance of recognizing pseudoasthma, the importance of timing of methacholine challenge, the usefulness of measuring the slope of the flow-volume curve, a goiter interfering with inspiratory flow, and several others. We also included several examples in which trend analyses of periodic pulmonary function tests were helpful.

The section on bronchial challenge was expanded to cover multiple-dose challenge. The volume exhaled in 6 seconds (FEV$_6$) is introduced as a surrogate for forced vital capacity in obstructive lung disease. Normal predicted values for the 6-minute walk test were added. Recent data from the Lung Health Study on the effect of weight gain on the forced vital capacity and forced expiratory volume in 1 second were included in the obesity section.

Robert E. Hyatt, M.D.
Paul D. Scanlon, M.D.
Masao Nakamura, M.D.

Acknowledgments

We thank Patricia A. Muldrow for typing this book. We appreciate the assistance of the Division of Media Support Services and of Kathryn J. Dolan in the Legal Department. Without the help of LeAnn Stee, Jane M. Craig, Kenna Atherton, and Roberta Schwartz in the Section of Scientific Publications this book would not have reached fruition.

List of Abbreviations

(A-a) D$_{O_2}$	difference between the oxygen tensions of alveolar gas and arterial blood
BMI	body mass index
Ca$_{O_2}$	arterial oxygen-carrying capacity
Ccw	chest wall compliance
C$_L$	compliance of the lung
C$_{L_{dyn}}$	dynamic compliance of the lung
C$_{L_{stat}}$	static compliance of the lung
COHb	carboxyhemoglobin
COPD	chronic obstructive pulmonary disease
Crs	static compliance of entire respiratory system
D$_L$	diffusing capacity of the lungs
D$_{L_{CO}}$	diffusing capacity of carbon monoxide
D$_{L_{O_2}}$	diffusing capacity of oxygen
ERV	expiratory reserve volume
FEF$_{25}$	forced expiratory flow after 25% of the FVC has been exhaled
FEF$_{25-75}$	forced expiratory flow over the middle 50% of the FVC
FEF$_{50}$	forced expiratory flow after 50% of the FVC has been exhaled
FEF$_{75}$	forced expiratory flow after 75% of the FVC has been exhaled
FEV$_1$	forced expiratory volume in 1 second
FEV$_6$	forced expiratory volume in 6 seconds
FEV$_1$/FVC	ratio of FEV$_1$ to the FVC
FIF$_{50}$	forced inspiratory flow after 50% of the VC has been inhaled
F$_{IO_2}$	fraction of inspired oxygen
FRC	functional residual capacity

FV	flow-volume
FVC	forced expiratory vital capacity
Hb	hemoglobin
MetHb	methemoglobin
MFSR	maximal flow static recoil (curve)
MIF	maximal inspiratory flow
MVV	maximal voluntary ventilation
Pa_{CO_2}	arterial carbon dioxide tension
Palv	alveolar pressure
Pao	pressure at the mouth
Pa_{O_2}	arterial oxygen tension
Patm	atmospheric pressure
P_{CO_2}	partial pressure of carbon dioxide
PEF	peak expiratory flow
PEmax	maximal expiratory pressure
PImax	maximal inspiratory pressure
P_{O_2}	partial pressure of oxygen
Ppl	pleural pressure
Pst	lung static elastic recoil pressure
PTLC	lung recoil pressure at TLC
Ptr	pressure inside the trachea
$P\bar{v}_{O_2}$	mixed venous oxygen tension
$\dot{Q}$	perfusion
R	resistance
Raw	airway resistance
Rpulm	pulmonary resistance
RV	residual volume
SAD	small airway disease
$SBD_{L_{CO}}$	single-breath method for estimating $D_{L_{CO}}$
SBN_2	single-breath nitrogen (test)
SVC	slow vital capacity
TLC	total lung capacity
$\dot{V}$	ventilation
V_A	alveolar volume
$\dot{V}_A$	alveolar ventilation
VC	vital capacity
$\dot{V}_{CO_2}$	carbon dioxide production
V_D	dead space volume
$\dot{V}_E$	ventilation measured at the mouth
$\dot{V}max$	maximal expiratory flow
$\dot{V}_{O_2}$	oxygen consumption

$\dot{V}_{O_2}max$	maximal oxygen consumption
$\dot{V}/\dot{Q}$	ventilation-perfusion
VR	ventilatory reserve
VT	tidal volume

1

Introduction

Pulmonary function tests are vastly underused, yet they can provide important clinical information. They are designed to identify and quantify defects and abnormalities in the function of the respiratory system and answer questions such as the following: How badly impaired is the patient's lung function? Is airway obstruction present? How severe is it? Does it respond to bronchodilators? Does the patient have impaired gas exchange? Is there impaired diffusion of oxygen from alveoli to pulmonary capillary blood? Is treatment helping the patient? How great is the surgical risk?

Pulmonary function tests can also answer other clinical questions: Is the patient's dyspnea due to cardiac or pulmonary dysfunction? Does the patient with chronic cough have occult asthma? Is obesity impairing the patient's pulmonary function? Is the patient's dyspnea due to weakness of the respiratory muscles?

The tests alone, however, cannot be expected to lead to a clinical diagnosis of, for example, pulmonary fibrosis or emphysema. Test results must be evaluated in light of the history; physical examination; chest radiograph; computed tomography scan, if available; and pertinent laboratory findings. Nevertheless, some test patterns strongly suggest the presence of certain conditions, such as pulmonary fibrosis. Also, the flow-volume loop associated with lesions of the trachea and upper airway is often so characteristic as to be nearly diagnostic of the presence of such a lesion (see Chapter 2).

As with any procedure, pulmonary function tests have shortcomings. There is some variability in the normal predicted values of various tests. In some studies, this variability is in part due to mixing asymptomatic smokers with nonsmokers in a "normal" population. Some variability is also seen among laboratories in the ways the tests are performed, the equipment is used, and the results are calculated.

This text assumes that the tests are performed accurately, and it focuses on their clinical significance. This approach is not to downplay the importance of the technician in obtaining accurate data. Procedures such as electrocardiography require relatively little technician training, especially with the new equipment that can detect errors such as faulty lead placement. And, of course, all the patient need do is lie still. In marked contrast is the considerable training required before a pulmonary function technician becomes "expert." With spirometry, for example, the patient must be exhorted to put forth maximal effort, and the technician must learn to detect submaximal effort. The patient is a very active participant in a number of the tests that are discussed here. Many of these tests have been likened to an athletic event—an apt analogy. In our experience, it takes several weeks of intense training before a technician becomes expert in administering common tests such as spirometry. If at all possible, the person interpreting the tests should undergo pulmonary function testing. Experiencing the tests is the best way to appreciate the challenges faced when administering the test to sick, often frightened patients.

However, the main problem with pulmonary function tests is that they are not ordered often enough. Population surveys generally document some abnormality in respiratory function in 5 to 20% of subjects studied. Chronic obstructive pulmonary disease (COPD) is currently the fourth leading cause of death in the United States. It causes more than 100,000 deaths per year. It is estimated that 16 million people in the United States currently have COPD. All too often the condition is not diagnosed until the disease is far advanced. In a significant number of cases, lung disease is still not being detected. If we are to make an impact on COPD, it needs to be detected early. Figure 1-1 shows the progression of a typical case of COPD. By the time dyspnea occurs, airway obstruction is moderately advanced. Looked at differently, spirometry can detect airway obstruction in COPD 5 to 10 years before dyspnea occurs.

Nevertheless, few physicians routinely order pulmonary function tests for their patients who smoke or for patients with mild to moderate dyspnea. For patients with dyspnea, however, in all likelihood the blood pressure has been checked and chest radiography and electrocardiography have been performed. We have

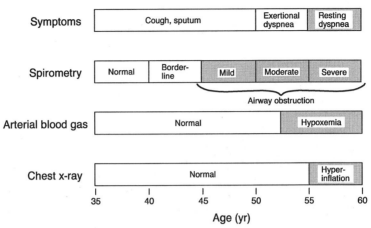

FIG. 1-1. Typical progression of the symptoms of chronic obstructive pulmonary disease (COPD). Only spirometry enables the detection of COPD years before shortness of breath develops. (From PL Enright, RE Hyatt [eds]: *Office Spirometry: A Practical Guide to the Selection and Use of Spirometers.* Philadelphia: Lea & Febiger, 1987. By permission of Mayo Foundation.)

seen patients who have had coronary angiography before simple spirometry identified the true cause of the patient's dyspnea.

Why are so few pulmonary function tests done? It is our impression that a great many clinicians are uncomfortable interpreting these tests. They are not sure what the tests measure or what they mean, and hence, the tests are not ordered. Unfortunately, very little time is devoted to this subject in medical school and in residency training. Furthermore, it is difficult to determine the practical clinical value of pulmonary function tests from currently available texts of pulmonary physiology and pulmonary function testing.

The sole purpose of, and justification for, this text is to make these tests user-friendly. Our goal is to target the basic clinical utility of the most common tests, which also happen to be the most important. Interesting but more complex procedures that have a less important clinical role are left to the standard physiologic texts.

2

Spirometry: Dynamic Lung Volumes

Spirometry is used to measure the rate at which the lung changes volume during forced breathing maneuvers. The most commonly performed test procedure uses the forced expiratory vital capacity (FVC) maneuver, in which the subject inhales maximally and then exhales as rapidly and completely as possible. Of all the tests considered in this book, the FVC test is the most important. Generally, it provides most of the information that is to be obtained from pulmonary function testing. It behooves the reader to have a thorough understanding of this procedure.

2A. SPIROGRAMS AND FLOW-VOLUME CURVE

The two methods of recording the FVC test are shown in Figure 2-1. In Figure 2-1A, the subject blows into a spirometer that records the volume exhaled, which is plotted as a function of time, the solid line. This is the classic spirogram showing the time course of a 4-L FVC. Two of the most common measurements made from this curve are the forced expiratory volume in 1 second (FEV_1) and the average forced expiratory flow rate over the middle 50% of the FVC (FEF_{25-75}). These are discussed later in this chapter.

The FVC test can also be plotted as a flow-volume (FV) curve, as in Figure 2-1B. The subject again exhales forcefully into the spirometer through a flowmeter that measures the flow rate (in liters per second) at which the subject exhales. The volume and the rapidity at which the volume is exhaled (flow in liters per second) are plotted as the FV curve. Several of the common measurements made from this curve are discussed later in this chapter.

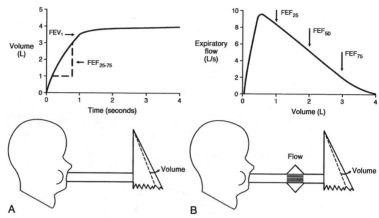

FIG. 2-1.   The two ways to record the forced vital capacity (FVC) maneuver. **A.** Volume recorded as a function of time, the spirogram. FEV_1, forced expiratory volume in 1 second; FEF_{25-75}, average forced expiratory flow rate over the middle 50% of the FVC. **B.** Flow recorded as a function of volume exhaled, the flow-volume curve. $FEF_{25(50,75)}$, forced expiratory flow after 25% (50%, 75%) of the FVC has been exhaled.

The two curves reflect the same data, and a computer can easily plot both curves with the subject exhaling through either a flowmeter or a volume recorder. Integration of flow provides volume, which, in turn, can be plotted as a function of time, and all the measurements shown in Figure 2-1 are also readily computed. Conversely, the volume signal can be differentiated with respect to time to determine flow. In our experience, *the ΓV representation (Fig. 2-1B) is the easiest to interpret and the most informative.* Therefore, we will use this representation almost exclusively.

Caution: It is extremely important that the subject be instructed and coached to perform the test properly. Expiration must be after a maximal inhalation, initiated as rapidly as possible, and continued with maximal effort until no more air can be expelled. "Good" and "bad" efforts are shown later on page 16 in Figure 2-6.

2B. VALUE OF THE FORCED EXPIRATORY VITAL CAPACITY TEST

The FVC test is the most important pulmonary function test for the following reason: For any given individual during expiration, there is a unique limit to the maximal flow that can be reached at any lung volume. This limit is reached with moderate expiratory efforts, and increasing the force used during expiration does not increase the flow. Consider in Figure 2-1B the maximal FV curve obtained from a normal subject during the FVC test. Once peak flow has been achieved, the rest of the curve defines the maximal flow that can be achieved at any lung volume. Thus, at FEF after 50% of the vital capacity has been exhaled (FEF_{50}), the subject cannot exceed a flow of 5.2 L/s regardless of how hard he or she tries. Note that the maximal flow that can be achieved decreases in an orderly fashion as more air is exhaled (that is, lung volume decreases) until at residual volume (4 L) no more air can be exhaled. The FVC test is so powerful because there is a limit to maximal expiratory flow at all lung volumes after 10 to 15% of FVC has been exhaled. Each individual has a unique maximal expiratory FV curve. Because this curve defines a limit to flow, the curve is highly reproducible in a given subject. Most important, maximal flow is very sensitive to the most common diseases that affect the lung.

The physics and aerodynamics causing this flow-limiting behavior are not explained here, but consider the simple lung model in Figure 2-2. A lung (a) is contained in a thorax (b) whose volume can be changed by the piston (c). Air from the lung exits the thorax via the trachea (d). The lung has elasticity, represented by the springs (e), and this elasticity is the major force expelling air from the lung. Elasticity also plays a major role in holding the compliant bronchi (f) open.

Figure 2-2A shows the lung at full inflation before a forced expiration. Figure 2-2B shows the lung during a forced expiration. As volume decreases, dynamic compression of the airway produces a critical narrowing that develops in the trachea and produces limitation of flow. As expiration continues and lung volume decreases even more, the narrowing migrates distally into the main bronchi and beyond. Three features of the model determine the maximal expiratory flow of the lung at any given lung volume: *lung elasticity* (e), which drives the flow and holds the airways open; *size* of the airways (f); and *resistance* to flow along these airways.

The great value of the FVC test is that it is very sensitive to diseases that alter the lung's mechanical properties:

1. In emphysema, lung tissue is lost (alveoli are destroyed), and elasticity is decreased. Airways are narrowed, flow

A. Full Inspiration

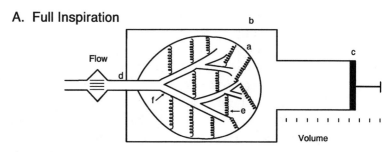

B. Forced Expiration

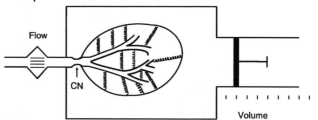

FIG. 2-2.   Simple lung model at full inflation (**A**) and during a forced deflation (**B**). The lung (a) is contained in a thorax (b) whose volume can be changed by the piston (c). Air exits from the lung via the trachea (d). The lung has elasticity (e), which both drives the flow and plays a role in holding the compliant bronchi (f) open. Critical narrowing (CN) occurs during the FVC maneuver.

resistance is increased, and both features lead to a decrease in maximal flow.

2. In chronic bronchitis, both mucosal thickening and thick secretions in the airways lead to airway narrowing, increased resistance to flow, and decreased maximal flow.

3. In asthma, the airways are narrowed as a result of bronchoconstriction and mucosal inflammation and edema. This narrowing increases resistance and decreases maximal flow.

4. In pulmonary fibrosis, the increased tissue elasticity may distend the airways and increase maximal flow, even though lung volume is reduced.

2C. NORMAL VALUES

There are tables and equations that are used to predict the normal values of the measurements to be discussed. The best values have been obtained from nonsmoking, normal subjects.

The important prediction variables are the size, sex, and age of the subject. Certain races, African American and Asian, for example, require race-specific values. Size is best estimated with body height. The taller the subject, the larger the lung and its airways, and thus maximal flows are higher. Women have smaller lungs than men of a given height. With aging, lung elasticity is lost, and thus airways are smaller and flows are lower. The inherent variability in normal predictive values must be kept in mind, however (as in the bell-shaped normal distribution curve of statistics). It is almost never known at what point in the normal distribution a given subject starts. For example, lung disease can develop in people with initially above-average lung volumes and flows. Despite a reduction from their initial baseline, they may still have values within the normal range of a population.

PEARL: Body height should not be used to estimate normal values for a subject with kyphoscoliosis. Why? Because the decreased height in such a subject will lead to a gross underestimation of the normal lung volume and flows. Rather the patient's arm span should be measured and used instead of height in the reference equations. In a 40-year-old man with kyphoscoliosis, vital capacity is predicted to be 2.78 L if his height of 147 cm is used, but the correct expected value of 5.18 L is predicted if his arm span of 178 cm is used—a 54% difference. The same principle applies to flow predictions.

2D. FORCED EXPIRATORY VITAL CAPACITY

The FVC is the volume expired during the FVC test; in Figure 2-1 the FVC is 4.0 L. Many abnormalities can cause a decrease in the FVC.

PEARL: To our knowledge, only one disorder, acromegaly, causes an abnormal *increase* in the FVC. The results of other tests of lung function are usually normal in this condition. However, persons with acromegaly are at increased risk for development of obstructive sleep apnea as a result of hypertrophy of the soft tissues of the upper airway.

Figure 2-3 presents a logical approach to considering possible causes of a decrease in FVC:

1. The problem may be with the *lung* itself. There may have been a resectional surgical procedure or areas of collapse.

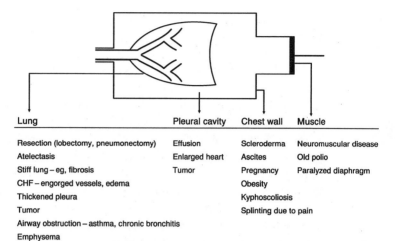

Lung	Pleural cavity	Chest wall	Muscle
Resection (lobectomy, pneumonectomy)	Effusion	Scleroderma	Neuromuscular disease
Atelectasis	Enlarged heart	Ascites	Old polio
Stiff lung – eg, fibrosis	Tumor	Pregnancy	Paralyzed diaphragm
CHF – engorged vessels, edema		Obesity	
Thickened pleura		Kyphoscoliosis	
Tumor		Splinting due to pain	
Airway obstruction – asthma, chronic bronchitis			
Emphysema			

FIG. 2-3.   Various conditions that can restrict the FVC. CHF, congestive heart failure.

Various other conditions can render the lung less expandable, such as fibrosis, congestive heart failure, and thickened pleura. Obstructive lung diseases may reduce the FVC by limiting deflation of the lung (Fig. 2-3).

2. The problem may be in the *pleural cavity*, such as an enlarged heart, pleural fluid, or a tumor encroaching on the lung.

3. Another possibility is restriction of the *chest wall*. The lung cannot inflate and deflate normally if the motion of the chest wall (which includes its abdominal components) is restricted.

4. Inflation and deflation of the system require normal function of the *respiratory muscles*, primarily the diaphragm, the intercostal muscles, and the abdominal muscles.

If the four possibilities listed are considered (lung, pleura, chest wall, muscles), the cause(s) of decreased FVC is usually determined. Of course, combinations of conditions occur, such as the enlarged failing heart with engorgement of the pulmonary vessels and pleural effusions. It should be remembered that the FVC is a maximally rapid expiratory vital capacity. The vital capacity may be larger when measured at slow flow rates; this situation is discussed in Chapter 3.

Two terms are frequently used in the interpretation of pulmonary function tests. One is an *obstructive defect*. This is lung disease that causes a decrease in maximal expiratory flow so that rapid emptying of the lungs is not possible; conditions such as emphysema, chronic bronchitis, and asthma cause this. Frequently, an associated decrease in the FVC occurs. A *restrictive defect* implies that lung volume, in this case the FVC, is reduced by any of the processes listed in Figure 2-3, *except* those causing obstruction.

Caution: In a restrictive process, the total lung capacity will be less than normal (see Chapter 3).

Earlier in the chapter it was noted that most alterations in lung mechanics lead to decreased maximal expiratory flows. Low expiratory flows due to airway obstruction are the hallmark of chronic bronchitis, emphysema, and asthma. The measurements commonly obtained to quantify expiratory obstruction are discussed below.

2E. FORCED EXPIRATORY VOLUME IN 1 SECOND

The FEV_1 is the most reproducible, most commonly obtained, and possibly most useful measurement. It is the volume of air exhaled in the first second of the FVC test. The normal value depends on the subject's size, age, sex, and race, just as does the FVC. Figure 2-4A and B show the FVC and FEV_1 from two normal subjects; the larger subject (A) has the bigger FVC and FEV_1.

When flow rates are slowed by airway obstruction, as in emphysema, the FEV_1 is decreased by an amount that reflects the severity of the disease. The FVC is also usually reduced, but to a lesser degree. Figure 2-4C shows a severe degree of obstruction. The 1-second volume (FEV_1) is easily identified directly from the spirogram. A 1-second mark can be added to the FV curve to identify the FEV_1, as shown in the figure. The common conditions producing expiratory slowing or obstruction are chronic bronchitis, emphysema, and asthma.

In Figure 2-4D, the FEV_1 is reduced because of a restrictive defect, such as pulmonary fibrosis. A logical question is, "How can I tell whether the FEV_1 is reduced as a result of airway obstruction or a restrictive process?" This question is considered next.

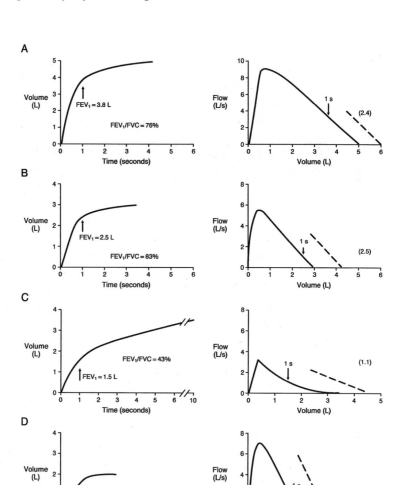

FIG. 2-4. Typical spirograms and flow-volume curves during forced expiration. **A** and **B** are from normal subjects of different sizes. **C** shows curves from a patient with severe airway obstruction, and **D** demonstrates curves typical of a pulmonary restrictive process. The arrows indicate the forced expiratory volume in 1 second (FEV$_1$). FEV$_1$/FVC ratios and the slopes of the flow-volume curves (dashed lines) are also shown.

2F. FEV$_1$/FVC RATIO

The FEV$_1$/FVC ratio is generally expressed as a percentage. The amount exhaled during the first second is a fairly constant fraction of the FVC, irrespective of lung size. In the normal adult, the ratio ranges from 75 to 85%, but it decreases somewhat with aging. Children have high flows for their size, and thus, their ratios are higher, up to 90%.

The significance of this ratio is twofold. First, it aids in quickly identifying persons with airway obstruction in whom the FVC is reduced. For example, in Figure 2-4C, the FEV$_1$/FVC is very low at 43%, indicating that the low FVC is due to airway obstruction and not pulmonary restriction. Second, the ratio is valuable for identifying the cause of a low FEV$_1$. In pulmonary restriction (without any associated obstruction), the FEV$_1$ and FVC are decreased proportionally; hence, the ratio is in the normal range, as in the case of fibrosis in Figure 2-4D, in which it is 87%. Indeed, in some cases of pulmonary fibrosis, the ratio may increase even more because of the increased elastic recoil of such a lung.

Thus, in regard to the question of how to determine whether airway obstruction or a restrictive process is causing a reduced FEV$_1$, the answer is to check the FEV$_1$/FVC ratio. A low FEV$_1$ with a normal ratio *usually* indicates a restrictive process, whereas a low FEV$_1$ and a decreased ratio signify a predominantly obstructive process.

In severe obstructive lung disease near the end of a forced expiration, the flows may be very low, barely perceptible. Continuation of the forced expiration can be very tiring and uncomfortable. To avoid patient fatigue, one can substitute the volume expired in 6 seconds, the FEV$_6$, for the FVC in the above ratio.

PEARL: Look at the FV curve. If significant scooping can be seen, as in Figure 2-4C, obstruction is present. In addition, look at the slope of the FV curve, the average change in flow divided by the change in volume. In normal subjects, this is roughly 2.5 (2.5 L/s per liter). The normal range is approximately 2.0 to 3.0. In the case of airway obstruction (Fig. 2-4C), the average slope is lower, 1.1. In the patient with fibrosis (Fig. 2-4D), the slope is normal to increased, 5.5. The *whole* curve needs to be studied.

Caution: Recall that a low FEV$_1$ and a normal FEV$_1$/FVC ratio *usually* indicate restriction. However, a subset of patients with

a low FEV_1 and normal FEV_1/FVC ratio also have a normal total lung capacity, which rules out significant restriction. This is
termed a "nonspecific ventilatory limitation" (see pages 37 and 38,
including Fig. 3-8).

2G. OTHER MEASURES OF MAXIMAL EXPIRATORY FLOW

Figure 2-5 shows the other most common measurements of maximal expiratory flow; they are all decreased in obstructive disease.

FEF_{25-75} is the average FEF rate over the middle 50% of the
FVC. This variable can be measured directly from the spirogram.
A microprocessor is used to obtain it from the FV curve. Some
investigators consider the FEF_{25-75} to be more sensitive than the
FEV_1 for detecting early airway obstruction, but it has a wider
range of normal values.

FEF_{50} is the flow after 50% of the FVC has been exhaled, and
FEF_{75} is the flow after 75% of the FVC has been exhaled.

Peak expiratory flow (PEF), which is also termed *maximal expiratory flow*, occurs shortly after the onset of expiration. It is reported in
either liters per minute or liters per second. The PEF, more than the
other measures, is very dependent on patient effort—the patient
must initially exhale as hard as possible to obtain reproducible
data. However, with practice, reproducible results are obtained.
Inexpensive portable devices allow patients to measure their PEF
at home and so monitor their status. This is particularly valuable
for patients with asthma.

As shown in Figure 2-5, these other measures, just as with the
FEV_1, can be reduced in the case of pure restrictive disease. Again,
the FV curve and the FEV_1/FVC ratio must be considered.

2H. HOW TO ESTIMATE PATIENT EFFORT
FROM THE FLOW-VOLUME CURVE

Although this text is not intended to consider test performance
(the results are assumed to be accurate), the FVC test must be
performed correctly. Generally, judgment about the performance
can be made from the FV curve. Occasionally, less than ideal
curves may be due to an underlying problem such as muscle
weakness.

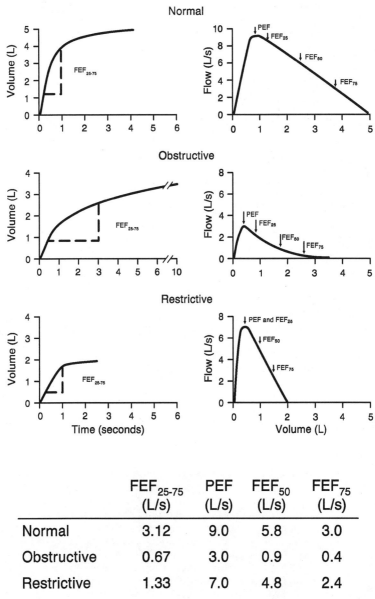

	FEF$_{25\text{-}75}$ (L/s)	PEF (L/s)	FEF$_{50}$ (L/s)	FEF$_{75}$ (L/s)
Normal	3.12	9.0	5.8	3.0
Obstructive	0.67	3.0	0.9	0.4
Restrictive	1.33	7.0	4.8	2.4

FIG. 2-5. Other measures of maximal expiratory flow in three typical conditions—normal, obstructive disease, and pulmonary restrictive disease. The average FEF rate over the middle 50% of the FVC (FEF$_{25\text{-}75}$) is obtained by measuring the volume exhaled over the middle portion of the FVC maneuvers and dividing it by the time required to exhale that volume. FEF$_{25}$, forced expiratory flow—flow after 25% of the FVC has been exhaled; FEF$_{50}$, flow after 50% of FVC has been exhaled; FEF$_{75}$, flow after 75% of FVC has been exhaled; PEF, peak expiratory flow.

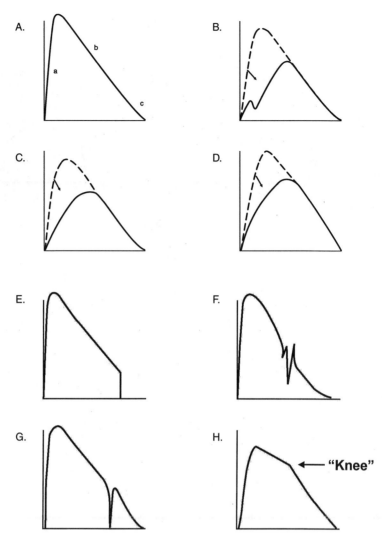

FIG. 2-6   Examples of good and unacceptable FVC maneuvers.
A. Excellent effort. a, rapid climb to peak flow; b, continuous decrease in
flow; c, termination at 0 to 0.1 L/s of zero flow. **B.** Hesitating start makes
curve unacceptable. **C.** Subject did not exert maximal effort at start of
expiration; test needs to be repeated. **D.** Such a curve almost always
indicates failure to exert maximal effort initially, but occasionally, it is
reproducible and valid, especially in young, nonsmoking females. This
is called a "rainbow curve." This curve may be found in children,
patients with neuromuscular disease, or subjects who perform the
maneuver poorly. In **B, C,** and **D,** the dashed line indicates the expected
curve; the *arrow* indicates the reduction in flow caused by performance
error. **E.** Curve shows good start, but subject quit too soon; test needs to
be repeated. Occasionally, this is reproducible, and this curve can be
normal for some young nonsmokers. **F.** Coughing during the first
second will decrease the FEV_1. The maneuver should be repeated.
G. Subject stopped exhaling momentarily; test needs to be repeated.
H. This curve with a "knee" is a normal variant that often is seen in
nonsmokers, especially young women.

In Figure 2-6, an excellent effort (*A*) is contrasted with ones that are unacceptable or require repeating of the test. The three features of the well-performed test are that (1) the curve shows a rapid climb to peak flow (a); (2) the curve then has a fairly smooth, continuous decrease in flow (b); and (3) the curve terminates at a flow within 0 to 0.1 L/s of zero flow or ideally at zero flow (c). The other curves in Figure 2-6 do not satisfy at least one of these features.

An additional important criterion is that the curves should be reproducible. Ideally, two curves should exhibit the above-described features and have peak flows within 10% of each other and FVC and FEV_1 volumes within 200 mL or 5% of each other. The technician needs to work with the patient to satisfy these reproducibility criteria. The physician must examine the selected curve for the contour characteristics. If the results are not satisfactory, the test needs to be repeated so that the data truly reflect the mechanical properties of a subject's lungs.

2I. MAXIMAL VOLUNTARY VENTILATION

The test for maximal voluntary ventilation (MVV) is an athletic event. The subject is instructed to breathe as *hard* and *fast* as possible for 10 to 15 seconds. The result is extrapolated to 60 seconds and reported in liters per minute. There can be a significant learning effect with this test, but a skilled technician can often avoid this problem.

A low MVV can occur in obstructive disease, in restrictive disease, in neuromuscular disease, in heart disease, in a patient who does not try or does not understand, or in a frail patient. Thus, this test is very nonspecific, and yet it correlates well with a subject's exercise capacity and with the complaint of dyspnea. It is also useful for estimating the subject's ability to withstand certain types of major operation (see Chapter 10).

PEARL: In a well-performed MVV test in a normal subject, the MVV is approximately equal to the FEV_1 x 40. If the FEV_1 is 3.0 L, the MVV should be approximately 120 L/min (40 x 3). On the basis of our experience and to be conservative, we set the lower limit of the predicted MVV at FEV_1 x 30. Example: A patient's FEV_1 is 2.5 L, and the MVV is 65 L/min. The FEV_1 x 30 product is 75 L/min, and thus, the MVV of 65 L/ min leads to a suspicion of poor effort, poor understanding, or fatigue. There are two important pathologic causes for the MVV to be less than the predicted lower limit: Obstructing lesions of the major airways (see section 2K, page 19) and respiratory muscle weakness (see section 9D, page 97). An MVV well in excess of this product may mean that the FEV_1 test was poorly performed. However, this product estimate may be less useful in advanced obstructive disease, when the subject's MVV sometimes exceeds that predicted from the FEV_1 (see case 20, Chapter 15, page 183).

PEARL: Some lesions of the major airway (see page 22, the Pearl) cause the MVV to be reduced out of proportion to the FEV_1. The same result can occur in patients who have muscle weakness, as in neuromuscular diseases (amyotrophic lateral sclerosis, myasthenia gravis, polymyositis). Thus, all these conditions need to be considered when the MVV is reduced out of proportion to the FEV_1.

2J. MAXIMAL INSPIRATORY FLOWS

With spirometer systems that measure both expiratory and inspiratory flows, the maximal inspiratory flow (MIF) can be measured. The usual approach is shown in Figure 2-7A. The subject exhales maximally (the FVC test) and then immediately inhales as rapidly and completely as possible, producing an inspiratory curve. The

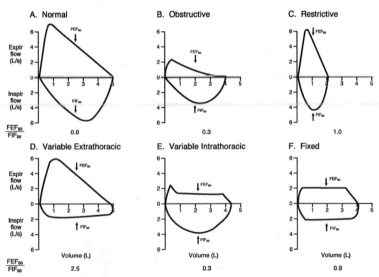

FIG. 2-7. Comparison of typical flow-volume loops (**A–C**) with the classic flow-volume loops in cases of lesions of the major airway (**D–F**). FEF_{50}, forced expiratory flow after 50% of the FVC has been exhaled; FIF_{50}, forced inspiratory flow measured at the same volume as FEF_{50}.

combined expiratory and inspiratory FV curves form the *FV loop*. Increased airway resistance decreases both maximal expiratory flow and MIF. However, unlike expiration, in which there is a limit to maximal flow, no mechanism such as dynamic compression limits MIF. Thus, it is very effort-dependent.

For these reasons, measurements of MIF are not widely obtained. They add little to the evaluation of the usual patient undergoing pulmonary function tests. The main value of testing MIF is for detecting lesions of the major airway.

2K. OBSTRUCTING LESIONS OF THE MAJOR AIRWAY

Obstructing lesions involving the major airway (carina to oral pharynx) are relatively uncommon. When present, however, they can often be detected by changes in the FV loop. This is a very important diagnosis to make.

The identification of these lesions from the FV loop depends on two characteristics. One is the *behavior* of the lesion during rapid expiration and inspiration. Does the lesion narrow and decrease flow excessively during one or the other phases of respiration? If it does, the lesion is categorized as *variable*. If the lesion is narrowed and decreases flow equally during both phases, the lesion is categorized as *fixed*. The other characteristic is the *location* of the lesion. Is it *extrathoracic* (above the thoracic outlet) or *intrathoracic* (to and including the carina but generally not beyond)?

Figure 2-7 illustrates typical FV loops in normal subjects (Fig. 2-7A), various disease states (Fig. 2-7B and C), and the three classic loops caused by lesions of the major airway (Fig. 2-7D–F). The factors that determine the unique contours of the curves for lesions of the major airway can be appreciated by considering the relationship between the intra-airway and extra-airway pressures during these forced maneuvers.

During *forced expiration*, the pressure inside the intrathoracic trachea (Ptr) is less than the surrounding pleural pressure (Ppl), and this airway region normally narrows. Outside the thorax, the airway pressure (Ptr) in the extrathoracic trachea is higher than the surrounding atmospheric pressure (Patm), and the region tends to stay distended. During *forced inspiration*, Ptr in the extrathoracic portion is lower than the surrounding pressure (that is, Patm), and therefore this region tends to narrow. In the intrathoracic trachea,

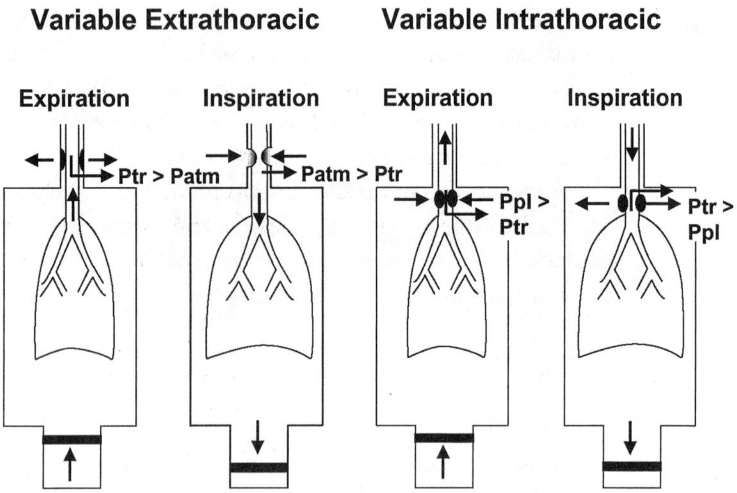

Variable Extrathoracic   Variable Intrathoracic

FIG. 2-8.   Model explaining the pathophysiology of the variable lesion of the major airway. Patm is the atmospheric pressure acting on the extrathoracic trachea. Ppl is the pressure in the pleural cavity that acts on the intrathoracic trachea. Ptr is the lateral, intratracheal airway pressure.

the surrounding Ppl is more negative than Ptr, which favors dilatation of this region. In the *variable* lesions, these normal changes in airway size are greatly exaggerated.

Figure 2-7D shows results with a *variable* lesion in the *extrathoracic* trachea. This may be caused by, for example, paralyzed but mobile vocal cords. This is explained by the model in Figure 2-8 (*left*). During expiration, the high intra-airway pressure (Ptr) keeps the cords distended and there may be little effect on expiratory flow. Ptr is greater than Patm acting on the outside of this lesion. During inspiration, however, the low pressure in the trachea causes marked narrowing of the cords with the remarkable reduction in flow seen in the inspiratory FV loop because Patm now greatly exceeds airway pressure, Ptr.

The model in Figure 2-8 (*right*) also explains Figure 2-7E, a *variable intrathoracic* lesion, for example, a compressible tracheal malignancy. During forced expiration, the high Ppl relative to airway pressure (Ptr) produces a marked narrowing with a dramatic constant reduction in expiratory flow in the FV loop. Yet inspiratory flow may be little affected because Ppl is more negative than airway pressure and the lesion distends.

Figure 2-7F shows the characteristic loop with a *fixed*, orifice-like lesion. Such a lesion—a napkin-ring cancer of the trachea or fixed, narrowed, paralyzed vocal cords—interferes almost equally with expiratory and inspiratory flows. The location of the lesion does not matter because the lesion does not change size regardless of the intra-airway and extra-airway pressures.

Various indices have been used to characterize these lesions of the major airway. Figure 2-7 shows the ratio of expiratory to inspiratory flow at 50% of the vital capacity (FEF_{50}/FIF_{50}). The ratio deviates most dramatically from the other curves in the variable lesion in the extrathoracic trachea (Fig. 2-7D). The ratio is nonspecific in the other lesions. The unique FV loop contours of the various lesions are the principal diagnostic features. Once a lesion of the major airway is suspected, confirmation by direct endoscopic visualization or radiographic imaging of the lesion is required.

Caution: Because some lesions may be predominantly, but not absolutely, variable or fixed, intermediate patterns can occur, but the loops are usually sufficiently abnormal to raise suspicion.

The spirograms corresponding to the lesions in Figure 2-7D through F are not shown because they are not nearly as useful as the FV loops for detecting these lesions. Some of the clinical situations in which we have encountered these abnormal FV loops are listed in Table 2-1.

TABLE 2-1. Examples of lesions of the major airway detected with the flow-volume loop

Variable extrathoracic lesions
    Vocal cord paralysis (due to thyroid operation, tumor invading
       recurrent laryngeal nerve, amyotrophic lateral sclerosis, post-polio)
    Subglottic stenosis
    Neoplasm (primary hypopharyngeal or tracheal, metastatic from
       primary lesion in lung or breast)
    Goiter
Variable intrathoracic lesions
    Tumor of lower trachea (below sternal notch)
    Tracheomalacia
    Strictures
    Wegener's granulomatosis or relapsing polychondritis
Fixed lesions
    Fixed neoplasm in central airway (at any level)
    Vocal cord paralysis with fixed stenosis
    Fibrotic stricture

PEARL: If an isolated, significant *decrease* in the MVV occurs in association with a normal FVC, FEV_1, and FEF_{25-75}, a major airway obstruction should be strongly suspected. A forced inspiratory vital capacity loop needs to be obtained. Not all laboratories routinely measure inspiratory loops. The technician needs to be asked whether stridor was heard during the MVV—it often is. In most such cases at our institution, these lesions are identified by technicians who find a low, unexplained MVV; may hear stridor; obtain the inspiratory loop; and hence make the diagnosis. Another consideration is whether the subject has a neuromuscular disorder, as discussed in section 9D, page 97.

2L. SMALL AIRWAY DISEASE

Small airway disease (SAD) is discussed here briefly primarily because the term has been used, but it is neither a particularly useful nor a necessarily proven concept.

The usefulness of the SAD concept hinges on two assumptions. First, usual chronic obstructive pulmonary disease (COPD) starts in the small (<2 mm diameter) peripheral airways. Second, there are specific pulmonary function tests that can detect early SAD.

As for the first assumption, there are questions as to whether peripheral airway disease presages clinical COPD. The second assumption led to the development of various tests as specific indicators of dysfunction of the small airway. None have proved to be particularly valuable, however. Tests such as density dependence of maximal expiratory flow and frequency dependence of compliance are difficult to perform and relatively nonspecific. (They are not discussed here. Chapter 8 discusses the closing volume—now out of favor—and the slope of phase III—a useful test.) The data that may best reflect peripheral airway function are the flows measured at low lung volumes during the FVC tests. These include the FEF_{25-75}, FEF_{50}, and FEF_{75} (see Fig. 2-5, page 15), but these tests do have a wide range of normal values.

2M. TYPICAL SPIROMETRIC PATTERNS

The typical test patterns discussed are summarized in Table 2-2. Because test results are nonspecific in lesions of the major airway, they are not included, the most diagnostically useful measure being the contour of the full FV loop.

TABLE 2-2. Typical patterns of impairment

Measurement	Obstructive	Restrictive
FVC (L)	N to ↓	↓
FEV$_1$ (L)	↓	↓
FEV$_1$/FVC (%)	N to ↓	N to ↑
FEF $_{25-75}$ (L/s)	↓	N to ↓
PEF (L/s)	↓	N to ↓
FEF$_{50}$ (L/s)	↓	N to ↓
Slope of FV curve	↓	↑
MVV (L/min)	↓	N to ↓

FEF$_{25-75}$, forced expiratory flow rate over the middle 50% of the FVC; FEF$_{50}$, forced expiratory flow after 50% of the FVC has been exhaled; FEV$_1$, forced expiratory volume in 1 second; FV, flow-volume; FVC, forced expiratory vital capacity; N, normal; PEF, peak expiratory flow; ↓, decreased; ↑, increased.
Comments:

1. If pulmonary fibrosis is suspected as the cause of restriction, diffusing capacity (see Chapter 4) and total lung capacity (see Chapter 3) should be determined.
2. If muscle weakness is suspected as a cause of restriction, maximal respiratory pressures should be determined (see Chapter 9).
3. For assessing the degree of emphysema, total lung capacity and diffusing capacity (see Chapters 3 and 4) should be determined.
4. If asthma is suspected, testing should be repeated after bronchodilator therapy (see Chapter 5).

2N. GESTALT APPROACH TO INTERPRETATION

Rather than merely memorizing patterns such as those listed in Table 2-2, another approach that is very useful is to visually compare the individual FV curve to the normal predicted curve (see Chapter 14).

In Figure 2-9A the dashed curve is the subject's normal, predicted FV curve. As a first approximation, this curve can be viewed as defining the maximal expiratory flows and volumes that can be achieved by the subject. In other words, it defines a mechanical limit to ventilation, and all expiratory flows are usually on or beneath the curve (that is, within the *area* under the curve).

Assume that COPD develops in the subject with the normal predicted curve in Figure 2-9A, and then the curve becomes that shown in Figure 2-9B. At a glance, this plot provides a lot of information. First, the subject has lost a great deal of the normal area (the shaded area) and is confined to breathing in the reduced area under the measured curve. Clearly, the subject has severe ventilatory limitation. The concave shape of the FV curve and the low

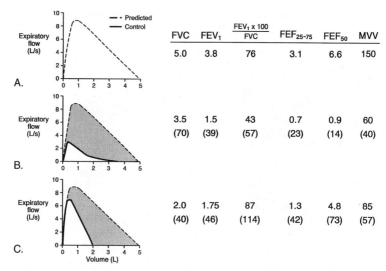

	FVC	FEV$_1$	$\dfrac{\text{FEV}_1 \times 100}{\text{FVC}}$	FEF$_{25-75}$	FEF$_{50}$	MVV
A.	5.0	3.8	76	3.1	6.6	150
B.	3.5	1.5	43	0.7	0.9	60
	(70)	(39)	(57)	(23)	(14)	(40)
C.	2.0	1.75	87	1.3	4.8	85
	(40)	(46)	(114)	(42)	(73)	(57)

FIG. 2-9. The gestalt approach to interpreting pulmonary function data when the predicted and observed flow-volume curves are available. The shaded area between the predicted and measured curves (**B** and **C**) provides a visual index of the degree of ventilatory limitation, there being none for the normal subject in **A**. **B** is typical of severe airway obstruction. **C** is typical of a severe pulmonary restrictive process. FEF$_{25-75}$, forced expiratory flow rate over the middle 50% of the FVC; FEF$_{50}$, forced expiratory flow after 50% of the FVC has been exhaled; FEV$_1$, forced expiratory volume in 1 second; FVC, forced vital capacity; MVV, maximal voluntary ventilation.

slope indicate an *obstructive* process. Before one even looks at the values to the right, it can be determined that the FVC and PEF are reduced and that the FEV$_1$, FEV$_1$/FVC ratio, FEF$_{25-75}$, and FEF$_{50}$ must also be reduced. Because the MVV is confined to this reduced area, it too will be decreased. The numbers in the figure confirm this.

Next, consider Figure 2-9C, in which the subject has interstitial pulmonary fibrosis. Again, a glance at the plot reveals that the subject has a substantial loss of area, indicating a moderately severe ventilatory limitation. The steep slope of the FV curve and the reduced FVC are consistent with the process being *restrictive*. A reduced FEV$_1$ but a normal FEV$_1$/FVC ratio can also be determined, and the flow rates (FEF$_{25-75}$ and FEF$_{50}$) can be expected to be normal to reduced. The MVV will be better preserved than shown in Figure 2-9B because high expiratory flows can still develop, albeit over a restricted volume range. The numbers confirm these conclusions.

The gestalt approach is a very useful first step in analyzing pulmonary function data. The degree of ventilatory limitation can be defined according to loss of area under the normal predicted FV curve, the shaded areas in Figure 2-9B and C. We arbitrarily define an area loss of 25% as a mild, 50% as a moderate, and 75% as a severe ventilatory limitation.

3

Static (Absolute) Lung Volumes

Measures of the so-called static (or absolute) lung volumes are often informative [1]. The most important are the vital capacity, residual volume, and total lung capacity. The *vital capacity (VC)* is measured by having the subject inhale maximally and then exhale *slowly* and completely. This VC is called the *slow vital capacity (SVC)*.

With complete exhaling, air still remains in the lung. This remaining volume is the *residual volume (RV)*. The RV can be visualized by comparing the inspiratory and expiratory chest radiographs (Fig. 3-1). The fact that the lungs do not collapse completely on full expiration is important physiologically. With complete collapse, transient hypoxemia would occur because mixed venous blood reaching the lung would have no oxygen to pick up. Furthermore, inflation of a collapsed lung requires very high inflating pressures, which would quickly fatigue the respiratory muscles and could tear the lung, leading to a *pneumothorax*. This is the problem in infants born with respiratory distress syndrome, in which portions of the lung can collapse (individual acinar units, up to whole lobes) at the end of exhalation. The RV can be measured and added to the SVC to obtain the *total lung capacity (TLC)*. Alternatively, the TLC can be measured and the SVC subtracted from it to obtain the RV. The value of these volumes is discussed on page 35.

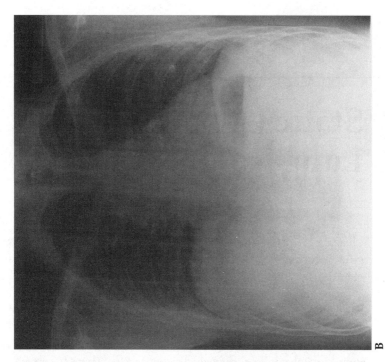

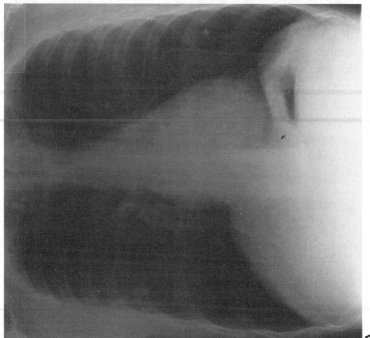

FIG. 3-1. Radiographs obtained from a normal subject at full inspiration (that is, at total lung capacity; **A**) and full expiration (**B**), in which the air remaining in the lung is the residual volume.

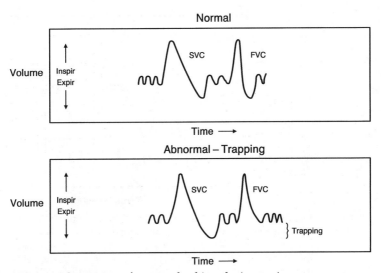

FIG. 3-2. Spirogram of a normal subject during various maneuvers compared with that of a subject with obstructive lung disease who shows "trapping." FVC, forced expiratory vital capacity; SVC, slow vital capacity.

3A. SLOW VITAL CAPACITY

Normally, the SVC and forced expiratory vital capacity (FVC; discussed in Chapter 2) are identical, as shown in the top panel of Figure 3-2. With airway obstruction, as in chronic obstructive pulmonary disease (COPD) or asthma, the FVC can be considerably smaller than the SVC, as shown in the lower panel of Figure 3-2. The difference between SVC and FVC reflects "trapping" of air in the lungs. The higher flows during the FVC maneuver cause excessive narrowing and closure of diseased airways in COPD, and thus the lung cannot empty as completely as during the SVC maneuver. Although "trapping" is of interest to the physiologist, it is of little value as a clinical measure. However, it does explain the possible discrepancies between the volumes of the SVC and the FVC.

3B. RESIDUAL VOLUME AND TOTAL LUNG CAPACITY

Figure 3-3 depicts the static lung volumes that are of most interest. The RV is measured (see page 31) and added to the SVC to obtain the TLC. The *expiratory reserve volume (ERV)* is the volume of air that

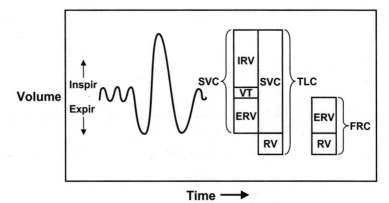

FIG. 3-3.   Various static (or absolute) lung volumes. Total lung capacity (TLC) is the sum of the residual volume (RV) and slow vital capacity (SVC). The SVC is the sum of the inspiratory reserve volume (IRV), the tidal volume (VT), and the expiratory reserve volume (ERV). The functional residual capacity (FRC) is the sum of the RV and the ERV.

can be exhaled after a normal expiration during quiet breathing (tidal breathing). The volume used during tidal breathing is the *tidal volume (VT)*. The *inspiratory reserve volume* is the volume of air that can be inhaled at the end of a normal tidal inspiration. The sum of the ERV and RV is termed the *functional residual capacity (FRC)*.

RV is the remaining volume of air in the lung at the end of a complete expiratory maneuver. It is determined by the limits of either the chest wall excursion or airway collapse or compression. In restrictive disorders, the limit of chest wall compression by the chest wall muscles determines RV. In obstructive disorders, the collapse of airways prevents air escape from the lungs, thereby determining the maximal amount exhaled. In obstructive disease, the RV is increased. The TLC is increased in most patients with chronic obstruction. However, TLC is often not increased in asthma. Finally, for a confident diagnosis of a *restrictive* process, the TLC must be *decreased*.

The FRC is primarily of interest to the physiologist. It is the lung volume at which the inward elastic recoil of the lung is balanced by the outward elastic forces of the relaxed chest wall (rib cage and abdomen). It is normally 40 to 50% of the TLC. When lung elasticity is reduced, as in emphysema, the FRC increases. It also increases to a lesser extent with normal aging. With the increased lung recoil in pulmonary fibrosis, the FRC decreases.

PEARL: The FRC is normally less when a subject is supine than when sitting or standing. When a person is upright, the heavy abdominal contents pull the relaxed diaphragm down, expanding both the rib cage and the lungs. In the supine position, gravity no longer pulls the abdominal contents downward; instead, the contents tend to push the diaphragm up, and thus the FRC is decreased. The lower FRC and hence, smaller lung volume in the supine position may interfere with gas exchange in patients with various types of lung disease and in the elderly. Blood drawn while these subjects are supine may show an abnormally low tension of oxygen in arterial blood. A similar effect often occurs in very obese subjects.

3C. HOW THE RESIDUAL VOLUME IS MEASURED

Usually, the FRC is measured by one of the methods to be described. If the ERV is subtracted from the FRC, the RV is obtained and, as noted previously, if the RV is added to the SVC, the TLC is obtained (Fig. 3-3).

As shown in Figure 3-2, the SVC may be larger than the FVC in obstructive disease. If the FVC is added to the RV, the TLC will be smaller than if the SVC is used. By convention, the SVC is used even in cases of COPD, in which there is often a considerable difference between the SVC and the FVC.

The three most commonly used methods of measuring the FRC (from which the RV is obtained) are nitrogen washout, inert gas dilution, and plethysmography. If these are not available, a radiographic method can be used.

Nitrogen Washout Method

The principle of this procedure is illustrated in Figure 3-4. At the end of a normal expiration, the patient is connected to the system. The lung contains an unknown volume (Vx) of air containing 80% nitrogen. With inspiration of nitrogen-free oxygen and exhalation into a separate bag, all the nitrogen can be washed out of the lung. The volume of the expired bag and its nitrogen concentration are measured, and the unknown volume is obtained with the simple mass balance equation. In practice, the procedure is terminated after 7 minutes and not all the nitrogen is removed from the lung, but this is easily corrected for. This procedure underestimates the FRC in patients with airway obstruction because in this condition there are lung regions that are very poorly

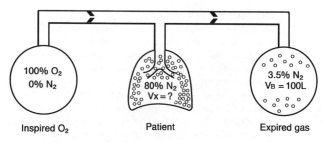

Initial volume of N_2 in patient = 0.8 (Vx)

Vx = FRC

Final volume of N_2 in expired bag = 0.035 (VB)

VB = volume of bag = 0.035 (100)

There is no loss of N_2 from system

so initial N_2 volume = final N_2 volume

0.8(Vx) = (0.035)(100)

Vx = 4.37 L = FRC

FIG. 3-4.   Nitrogen washout method of measuring the functional residual capacity (FRC). The initial volume of nitrogen (N_2) in the lungs at FRC equals 80% N_2 × FRC volume. The N_2 volume of the inhaled oxygen (O_2) is zero. The volume of N_2 washed out of the lung is computed as shown, and the FRC, or Vx, is obtained by solving the mass balance equation, 0.8 (Vx) = 0.035 (VB).

ventilated, and hence, they lose very little of their nitrogen. A truer estimate in obstructive disease can be obtained if this test is prolonged to 15 to 20 minutes. However, patients then find the test unpleasant.

Inert Gas Dilution Technique

The concept is illustrated in Figure 3-5. Helium, argon, or neon can be used. The spirometer system contains a known volume of gas (V1), (in Fig. 3-5 it is helium with a known concentration, C_1.) At FRC, the subject is connected to the system and rebreathes until the helium concentration reaches a plateau indicating equal concentrations of helium (C_2) in the spirometer and lung. Because essentially no helium is absorbed, Equations 1 and 2 can be combined and solved for Vx, the FRC. In practice, oxygen is added to the circuit to replace that consumed by the subject, and carbon dioxide is absorbed to prevent hypercarbia. As with the nitrogen washout technique, the gas dilution method underestimates the FRC in patients with airway obstruction.

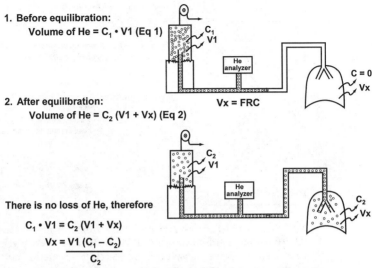

1. Before equilibration:
Volume of He = $C_1 \cdot V1$ (Eq 1)

2. After equilibration:
Volume of He = $C_2 (V1 + Vx)$ (Eq 2)

There is no loss of He, therefore

$$C_1 \cdot V1 = C_2 (V1 + Vx)$$

$$Vx = \frac{V1 (C_1 - C_2)}{C_2}$$

FIG. 3-5. Helium dilution technique of measuring the functional residual capacity (FRC). Before the test, no helium (He) is present in the lungs (Vx), and there is a known volume of He in the spirometer and tubing—the concentration of He (C_1) times the volume of the spirometer and the connecting tubes (V1). At equilibrium, the concentration of He (C_2) is uniform throughout the system. The mass balance equation can now be solved for the FRC (Vx).

Plethysmography

The principle of plethysmography is simple. The theory is based on Boyle's law, which states that the product of the pressure (P) and volume (V) (PV) of a gas is constant under constant temperature (isothermal) conditions. The gas in the lungs is isothermal because of its intimate contact with capillary blood. The technique is shown in Figure 3-6 with the standard constant-volume body plethysmograph. An attractive feature of this technique is that several measurements of RV and TLC can be obtained quickly. This is not possible with the washout and dilution methods because the alveolar gas composition must be brought back to the control state before these tests can be repeated, a process that often takes 10 to 20 minutes in patients with COPD. The plethysmographic method measures essentially all the gas in the lung, including that in poorly ventilated areas. Thus, in COPD, the FRC, RV, and TLC obtained with this method are usually larger and more accurate than those with the gas methods. Often the TLC of a patient with COPD is 2 to 3 L more with plethysmography.

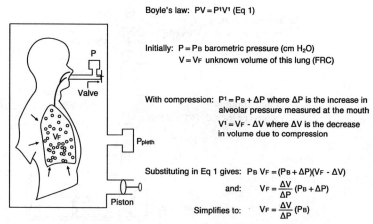

Boyle's law: $PV = P^1V^1$ (Eq 1)

Initially: $P = P_B$ barometric pressure (cm H_2O)
$V = V_F$ unknown volume of this lung (FRC)

With compression: $P^1 = P_B + \Delta P$ where ΔP is the increase in alveolar pressure measured at the mouth

$V^1 = V_F - \Delta V$ where ΔV is the decrease in volume due to compression

Substituting in Eq 1 gives: $P_B V_F = (P_B + \Delta P)(V_F - \Delta V)$

and: $V_F = \dfrac{\Delta V}{\Delta P} (P_B + \Delta P)$

Simplifies to: $V_F = \dfrac{\Delta V}{\Delta P} (P_B)$

FIG. 3-6. The equipment and the measurements needed to measure the functional residual capacity (FRC) by using a body plethysmograph and applying Boyle's law (Eq 1). The subject is seated in an airtight plethysmograph and the pressure in the plethysmograph (Ppleth) changes with changes in lung volume. When the subject stops breathing, alveolar pressure equals barometric pressure (Pb). Consider what happens if the valve at the mouth is closed at the end of a quiet expiration, i.e., FRC, and the subject makes an expiratory effort. Alveolar pressure increases by an amount (ΔP) that is measured by the mouth gauge, P. Lung volume decreases as a result of gas compression, there being no airflow, and hence Ppleth decreases. The change in Ppleth provides a measure of the change in volume (ΔV), as follows. With the subject momentarily not breathing, the piston pump is cycled and the known volume changes produce known changes in Ppleth. These measurements provide all the data needed to solve the above equation for V_F. The final equation is simplified by omitting ΔP from the quantity ($P_B + \Delta P$). Because ΔP is small (~ 20 cm H_2O) compared with P_B ($\sim 1,000$ cm H_2O), it can be neglected. PV, product of pressure and volume.

Radiographic Method

If the above-described methods are not available, radiographic methods can provide a good estimate of TLC. Posterior-anterior and lateral radiographs are obtained while the subject holds his or her breath at TLC. TLC is estimated by either planimetry or the elliptic method [2]. The radiographic technique compares favorably with the body plethysmographic method and is more accurate than the gas methods in subjects with COPD. It is also accurate in patients with pulmonary fibrosis. The technique is not difficult but requires that radiographs be obtained at maximal inspiration.

3D. SIGNIFICANCE OF RESIDUAL VOLUME
AND TOTAL LUNG CAPACITY

Knowledge of the RV and TLC can help in determining whether a restrictive or an obstructive process is the cause of a decrease in FVC and forced expiratory volume in 1 second (FEV_1). This distinction is not always apparent from the flow-volume (FV) curves. The chest radiographs may help when obvious hyperinflation or fibrosis is present.

As noted in section 2F, page 13, the (FEV_1)/FVC ratio usually provides the answer. However, in a patient with asthma who is not wheezing and has a decreased FVC and (FEV_1), both the (FEV_1)/FVC ratio and the slope of the FV curve may be normal. In this case the RV should be mildly increased, but often the TLC is normal.

The TLC and RV are increased in COPD, especially emphysema. Usually the RV is increased more than the TLC, and thus the RV/TLC ratio is also increased. The TLC and RV are also increased in acromegaly, but the RV/TLC ratio is normal.

By definition, the TLC is reduced in restrictive disease, and usually the RV is also reduced. The diagnosis of a restrictive process cannot be made with confidence unless there is evidence of a decreased TLC. The evidence may be the direct measure of TLC or the apparent volume reduction seen on the chest radiograph, or it may be suggested by the presence of a very steep slope of the FV curve (see Fig. 2-4).

PEARL: Lung resection for lung cancer or bronchiectasis decreases the RV and TLC, but this is an unusual restrictive process. Because there is often associated airway obstruction, the RV/TLC may be abnormally high. Furthermore, an obstructive process will be apparent because of the shape of the FV curve and a decreased (FEV_1)/FVC ratio. This is a mixed restrictive-obstructive pattern.

3E. EXPANDING THE GESTALT APPROACH
TO ABSOLUTE LUNG VOLUME DATA

Figure 3-7 shows the FV curves from Figure 2-9 as a means to consider what changes might be expected in the absolute lung

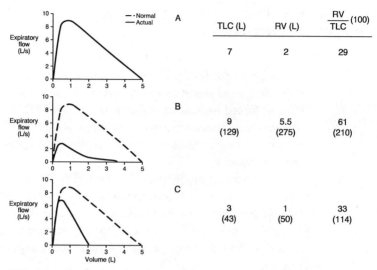

FIG. 3-7.   Further application of the gestalt approach introduced in Figure 2-9, page 24. Note that the area between the predicted (dashed line) and observed (solid line) flow-volume curves is not shaded. **A.** Normal pattern. **B.** Severe obstruction. **C.** Severe pulmonary restriction. (The numbers in parentheses are the percentage of predicted normal.) RV, residual volume; TLC, total lung capacity.

volumes. Figure 3-7*A* represents findings in a normal subject: TLC of 7 L, RV of 2 L, and RV/TLC ratio of 29%.

Figure 3-7*B* shows a severe ventilatory limitation due to airway obstruction. In addition to the reduced flows, TLC and RV are expected to be increased, RV more than TLC, so that the RV/TLC ratio will also be abnormal. These expectations are confirmed by the values on the right of the figure. However, the effect of lung resection in COPD needs to be considered (see section 3D).

The FV curve in Figure 3-7*C* is consistent with severe ventilatory limitation due to a restrictive process. This diagnosis requires the TLC to be decreased, and the RV/TLC ratio is expected to be essentially normal. The values on the right of the figure confirm these expectations.

A question in regard to Figure 3-7*C* is, What is the cause of this restrictive process? The answer to this question requires review of Figure 2-3 (page 10), in which all but the obstructive diseases need to be considered. Most restrictive processes can be evaluated from the history, physical examination, and chest radiograph. In fibrosis, diffusing capacity (discussed in Chapter 4) is expected to be reduced and radiographic changes evident. Poor patient effort can be *excluded* by evaluating the FV curve (see Fig. 2-6, page 16) and by noting that the patient gives reproducible efforts.

A curve similar to that in Figure 3-7C but with reduced peak flows is found in patients with normal lungs in whom a neuromuscular disorder such as amyotrophic lateral sclerosis or muscular dystrophy develops. In this case, the maximal voluntary ventilation is often reduced (see section 2I, page 17). In addition, with this reduction in the FVC, the maximal respiratory muscle strength is reduced, as discussed in Chapter 9. Interestingly, patients with bilateral diaphragmatic paralysis can present with this pattern. However, these patients differ in that their dyspnea becomes extreme, and often intolerable, when they lie down.

Some massively obese subjects also show the pattern in Figure 3-7C. They have a very abnormal ratio of weight (in kilograms) to height (in centimeters). Normally, this ratio is less than 0.5. In massively obese subjects it is often greater than 0.75. In recent years, body mass index (BMI) has become the standard index for obesity. It is body weight (in kilograms) divided by height (in meters, squared): kg/m^2. In general, a BMI more than 28 is overweight. Extremes of obesity range above 50 to 70 or more. In our laboratory, we find that a BMI more than 35 is associated with an average reduction in FVC of 5 to 10% (unpublished data). There is a large variation, however: Some obese individuals have normal lung volumes, and others are more severely affected. This difference may be related to fat distribution or to the relationship between fat mass and muscular mass [3].

Figure 3-8 shows two curves in which the FEV_1 and FVC are reduced and the FEV_1/FVC ratio is normal. Both are *consistent* with a restrictive process. However, in both cases the TLC is normal. Therefore, the diagnosis of a restrictive process *cannot* be made. In this case, the term "nonspecific ventilatory limitation" is applied (see section 2F, page 13).

Sometimes a more definitive diagnosis can be made. For example, Figure 3-8A shows a parallel shift of the FV curve. Ventilatory limitation is mild to moderate. This finding is common in mild asthma. The TLC is normal, and the RV and RV/TLC are only mildly increased. The history may be consistent with asthma with or without wheezing. The subject often has a higher than normal

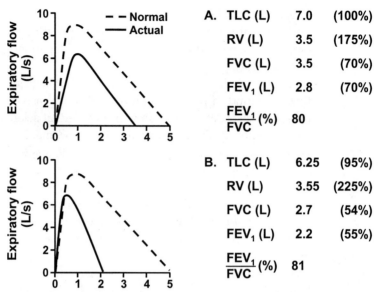

A.	TLC (L)	7.0	(100%)
	RV (L)	3.5	(175%)
	FVC (L)	3.5	(70%)
	FEV$_1$ (L)	2.8	(70%)
	$\dfrac{\text{FEV}_1}{\text{FVC}}$ (%)	80	

B.	TLC (L)	6.25	(95%)
	RV (L)	3.55	(225%)
	FVC (L)	2.7	(54%)
	FEV$_1$ (L)	2.2	(55%)
	$\dfrac{\text{FEV}_1}{\text{FVC}}$ (%)	81	

FIG. 3-8.   **A** and **B**. Examples of nonspecific ventilatory impairment in which the forced expiratory volume in 1 second (FEV$_1$) and forced expiratory vital capacity (FVC) are reduced proportionately, giving a normal FEV$_1$/FVC ratio, and the total lung capacity (TLC) is normal. The numbers in parentheses are the percentage of predicted normal. Note that residual volume (RV) is increased. This should not be confused with obstructive disorders in which RV is also increased.

increase in expiratory flows on the FV curve after use of an inhaled bronchodilator. If this does not occur, a methacholine challenge test is often recommended in an attempt to uncover a possible asthmatic process. These procedures are discussed in Chapter 5.

Figure 3-8B is a nonspecific ventilatory limitation of moderate degree. In this case, the slope of the FV curve is increased and not normal, but there is no clinical evidence of parenchymal involvement, and the pulmonary diffusing capacity (D$_\text{LCO}$, see Chapter 4) is normal. This pattern can occur in patients with relatively quiescent asthma. A thorough history and physical examination may uncover the problem. The response to a bronchodilator may be marked, or results of the methacholine challenge test may be positive. Also, some obese subjects have a normal TLC and the pattern shown in Figure 3-8B instead of the pattern in Figure 3-7C.

We have studied charts of 21 patients in whom there was a nonspecific ventilatory limitation with normal TLC and D$_\text{LCO}$. In 38% the patients had obesity alone ($n = 3$), asthma alone ($n = 1$), or

TABLE 3-1. Typical patterns of impairment

Measurement	Obstructive	Restrictive
FVC (L)	↓	↓
FEV$_1$ (L)	↓	↓
FEV$_1$/FVC (%)	N to ↓	N to ↑
FEF$_{25-75}$ (L/s)	↓	N to ↓
PEF (L/s)	↓	N to ↓
FEF$_{50}$ (L/s)	↓	N to ↓
Slope of FV curve	↓	↑
MVV (L/min)	↓	N to ↓
TLC	N to ↑	↓
RV	↑	↓
RV/TLC (%)	↑	N

FEF$_{25-75}$, forced expiratory flow rate over the middle 50% of the FVC; FEF$_{50}$, forced expiratory flow after 50% of the FVC has been exhaled; FEV$_1$, forced expiratory volume in 1 second; FV, flow-volume; FVC, forced expiratory vital capacity; MVV, maximal voluntary ventilation; N, normal; PEF, peak expiratory flow; RV, residual volume; TLC, total lung capacity; ↓, decreased; ↑, increased.

asthma and obesity ($n = 4$). The mean weight:height ratios were 0.66, 0.53, and 0.67 for obesity, asthma, and asthma and obesity, respectively. In 29% there was a mild parenchymal infiltrate ($n = 6$), and 33% were normal ($n = 3$) or had an uncertain diagnosis ($n = 4$). The seven cases that were normal or had an uncertain diagnosis are classified as nonspecific ventilatory limitation. Possibly this is a normal variant. Other possibilities are early undetectable pulmonary fibrosis or an interaction of aging and moderate obesity. Often, however, there is no clue. Normal predicted values of the FV curves are relied on heavily. The values used in our laboratory are given in the Appendix.

Table 3-1 is an expansion of Table 2-2 (page 23): The TLC, RV, and RV/TLC ratio are added.

PEARL: Assume you had estimates of TLC by the plethysmographic method and the dilution methods (nitrogen or helium). If the plethysmographic TLC exceeds that of the dilution method, you have an estimate of the volume of poorly ventilated lung, which is characteristic of airway obstruction. In section 4C, page 43, another estimate of poorly ventilated volume is described when the D$_{LCO}$ is measured.

PEARL: What determines RV? As normal adults exhale slowly and completely, airway resistance increases dramatically at very low volumes as the airways narrow (see Fig. 7-4, page 78). When airway resistance approaches infinity, no further exhalation occurs and RV is reached. At this point, the small, peripheral airways are essentially closed. An increase in RV is sometimes the first sign of early airway disease. An interesting exception to this description of how RV in adults is determined can occur in children and young adults. Their FV curve shows an abrupt cessation of flow with a contour similar to that seen in Figure 2-6E (page 16). An increase in airway resistance does not cause exhalation to cease. Rather, the respiratory muscles are not strong enough to compress the chest wall and abdomen any further. This increase in RV is not abnormal and usually disappears with aging.

REFERENCES

1. Gibson GJ. Lung volumes and elasticity. *Clin Chest Med* 22:623–635, 2001.
2. Miller RD, Offord KP. Roentgenologic determination of total lung capacity. *Mayo Clin Proc* 55: 694–699, 1980.
3. Cotes JE, Chinn DJ, Reed JW. Body mass, fat percentage, and fat free mass as reference variables for lung function: effects on terms for age and sex. *Thorax* 56:839–844, 2001.

4

Diffusing Capacity
of the Lungs

An important step in the transfer of oxygen from ambient air to the arterial blood is the process of diffusion, that is, the transfer of oxygen from the alveolar gas to the hemoglobin within the red cell. The pertinent anatomy is shown in Figure 4-1A. The path taken by oxygen molecules is shown in Figure 4-1B. They must traverse the alveolar wall, capillary wall, plasma, and red cell membrane and then combine with hemoglobin.

4A. THE DIFFUSING CAPACITY OF THE LUNGS

The diffusing capacity of the lungs (D_L) estimates the transfer of oxygen from alveolar gas to red cell. The amount of oxygen transferred is largely determined by three factors. One factor is the *area* (*A*) of the alveolar-capillary membrane, which consists of the alveolar and capillary walls. The greater the area, the greater the rate of transfer and the higher the D_L. Area is influenced by the number of blood-containing capillaries in the alveolar wall. The second factor is the *thickness* (*T*) of the membrane. The thicker the membrane, the lower the D_L. The third factor is the *driving pressure*, that is, the difference in oxygen tension between the alveolar gas and the venous blood (ΔP_{O_2}). Alveolar oxygen tension is higher than that in the deoxygenated venous blood of the pulmonary artery. The greater this difference (ΔP_{O_2}), the more oxygen transferred. These relations can be expressed as

$$D_L \cong \frac{A \times \Delta P_{O_2}}{T}$$

(Eq. 1)

41

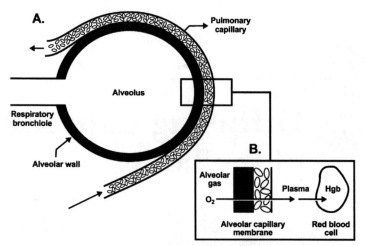

FIG. 4-1.   Alveolar-capillary membrane through which oxygen must diffuse to enter the blood. In **B,** alveolar wall is represented by the black rectangle. Hgb, hemoglobin.

4B. THE DIFFUSING CAPACITY FOR CARBON MONOXIDE

The diffusing capacity of oxygen (DL_{O_2}) can be measured directly, but this is technically extremely difficult. Measuring the diffusing capacity of carbon monoxide (DL_{CO}) is much easier and provides a valid reflection of the diffusion of oxygen. In essence, carbon monoxide is substituted for oxygen in Equation 1.

Several techniques for estimating DL_{CO} have been described. The most widely used is the single-breath (SB) method ($SBDL_{CO}$). The subject exhales to residual volume and then inhales a gas mixture containing a very low concentration of carbon monoxide plus an inert gas, usually helium. After a maximal inhalation to total lung capacity (TLC), the subject holds his or her breath for 10 seconds and then exhales completely. A sample of exhaled alveolar gas is collected and analyzed. By measuring the concentration of the exhaled carbon monoxide and helium, the value of the DL_{CO} can be computed. The helium is used to calculate TLC, and the exhaled carbon monoxide is used to calculate the amount of carbon monoxide transferred to the blood.

The technical details of measurement of $SBDL_{CO}$ are complex. To improve accuracy and reproducibility of testing among laboratories, the American Thoracic Society has established standards for performance of the test [1,2].

4C. NORMAL VALUES OF $D_{L_{CO}}$

An average normal value is 20 to 30 mL/min per mm Hg; that is, 20 to 30 mL carbon monoxide is transferred per minute per mm Hg difference in the driving pressure of carbon monoxide. The normal values depend on age (decrease with aging), sex (slightly lower in females), and size (taller people have larger lungs and therefore a higher $D_{L_{CO}}$). The inclusion of helium provides an estimate of total alveolar volume (V_A). Dividing $D_{L_{CO}}$ by V_A tends to normalize for difference in size and therefore the $D_{L_{CO}}/V_A$ ratio (or Krogh constant) tends to be the same in various-sized normal subjects. To an extent in a given subject, the $D_{L_{CO}}$ is also directly related to the volume of the inhaled breath. The smaller the volume, the lower the $D_{L_{CO}}$. The $D_{L_{CO}}/V_A$ in this situation would change little, however, if at all. This fact is useful, especially when repeated tests are obtained over time. The volume inhaled might vary from year to year, but the $D_{L_{CO}}/V_A$ tends to correct for this. Most patients can hold their breath for 10 seconds, but some subjects with very small vital capacities cannot inhale a sufficient quantity of the gas mixture to give a valid test.

> **PEARL:** In the normal subject, the V_A is essentially the same as the TLC and can be used as an estimate of TLC. With obstructive disease, V_A underestimates TLC, just as the nitrogen washout and inert gas dilution techniques do (see section 3C, page 31). However, TLC obtained with plethysmography minus the V_A provides an estimate of the severity of nonuniform gas distribution, i.e., the volume of poorly ventilated lung (see first Pearl, page 39).

4D. CAUSES OF INCREASED $D_{L_{CO}}$

Usually, an increased $D_{L_{CO}}$ is not a concern. However, there are some interesting causes of an increased $D_{L_{CO}}$, as follows:

1. Supine position: Rarely is the $D_{L_{CO}}$ measured while the subject is supine, but this position produces a higher value because of increased perfusion and blood volume of the upper lobes.
2. Exercise: It is difficult to hold one's breath for 10 seconds during exercise. When this is done just after exercise, however, $D_{L_{CO}}$ is increased because of increased pulmonary blood volumes.

3. Asthma: Some patients with asthma, especially when symptom-free, have an increased D_{LCO}, possibly because of more uniform distribution of pulmonary blood flow.

4. Obesity: The D_{LCO} can be increased in obese persons, especially those who are massively obese. This increase is thought to be due to an increased pulmonary blood volume.

5. Polycythemia: This is an increase in capillary red cell mass. This essentially amounts to an increase in area (A) in Equation 1.

6. Intra-alveolar hemorrhage: In conditions such as Goodpasture's syndrome, the hemoglobin in the alveoli combines with carbon monoxide to produce an artificially high uptake of carbon monoxide, which causes an increase in the calculated D_{LCO}. Indeed, sequential D_{LCO} measurements have been used to follow increases or decreases in intra-alveolar hemorrhage.

7. Left-to-right intracardiac shunts: These lead to an increased pulmonary capillary volume.

4E. CAUSES OF DECREASED D_{LCO}

Any process that decreases the surface area available for diffusion or thickens the alveolar-capillary membrane will decrease the D_{LCO} (Fig. 4-1B and Eq. 1). On the basis of these considerations, conditions that reduce the diffusing capacity can be determined (Table 4-1). The major ones are listed here.

Conditions That Decrease Surface Area

1. Emphysema: Although lung volume is increased, alveolar walls and capillaries are destroyed, and thus, the total surface area is reduced. Reduction of the D_{LCO} in a patient with significant airway obstruction strongly suggests underlying emphysema.

2. Lung resection: If only a small portion of lung is resected (such as a lobe in an otherwise normal patient), capillary recruitment from the remaining normal lung can result in an unchanged D_{LCO}. If sufficient capillary surface area is lost, as with a pneumonectomy, the D_{LCO} is reduced.

TABLE 4-1. Causes of a decreased diffusing capacity

Decreased *area* for diffusion
  Emphysema
  Lung/lobe resection
  Bronchial obstruction, as by tumor
  Multiple pulmonary emboli
  Anemia
Increased *thickness* of alveolar-capillary membrane
  Idiopathic pulmonary fibrosis
  Congestive heart failure
  Asbestosis
  Sarcoidosis, involving parenchyma
  Collagen vascular disease—scleroderma, systemic lupus
    erythematosus
  Drug-induced alveolitis or fibrosis—bleomycin, nitrofurantoin,
    amiodarone, methotrexate
  Hypersensitivity pneumonitis, including farmer's lung
  Histiocytosis X (eosinophilic granuloma)
  Alveolar proteinosis
Miscellanous
  High carbon monoxide back pressure from smoking
  Pregnancy
  Ventilation-perfusion mismatch

3. Bronchial obstruction: A tumor obstructing a bronchus obviously reduces area and lung volume. Again, the D_{LCO}/V_A might be normal.

4. Multiple pulmonary emboli: By blocking perfusion to alveolar capillaries, emboli effectively reduce area. Also, primary pulmonary hypertension causes a reduction in capillary area.

5. Anemia: By reducing pulmonary capillary hemoglobin, anemia also effectively reduces area, as does any condition that lowers capillary blood volume. The usual correction for men with anemia is this equation:

$$D_{LCO}\,(cor) = D_{LCO}\,(unc) \times [10.22 + Hb]/[1.7 \times Hb] \qquad (Eq.\ 2)\ [1]$$

where cor is corrected, unc is uncorrected, and Hb is hemoglobin. For women, the factor in the first set of brackets is 9.38 instead of 10.22.

Conditions That Effectively Increase Wall Thickness

As is discussed in Chapter 6, however, much of the reduction in DL_{CO} in these fibrotic conditions is thought to be due to mismatching of ventilation and perfusion.

1. Idiopathic pulmonary fibrosis: This is also called cryptogenic fibrosing alveolitis. It thickens the alveolar-capillary membrane and also decreases lung volume.
2. Congestive heart failure: In this disorder, transudation of fluid into the interstitial space (tissue edema) or into the alveoli lengthens the pathway for diffusion.
3. Asbestosis: This is pulmonary fibrosis caused by exposure to asbestos.
4. Sarcoidosis: This involves the lung parenchyma.
5. Collagen vascular disease: Conditions such as scleroderma and systemic lupus erythematosus probably alter or obliterate capillary walls, a situation that effectively increases the barrier to diffusion. This may be the first pulmonary function test to become abnormal in these conditions.
6. Drug-induced alveolitis or fibrosis: Bleomycin, nitrofurantoin, amiodarone, and methotrexate can be involved in these conditions.
7. Hypersensitivity pneumonitis: This condition includes farmer's lung.
8. Histiocytosis X: This condition is eosinophilic granuloma of the lung or Langerhans' cell histiocytosis.
9. Alveolar proteinosis: Alveoli are filled with a phospholipid-rich material.

Miscellaneous Causes

1. The high carbon monoxide tension in the blood of a heavy smoker can decrease the ΔP_{CO} or driving pressure. This lowers the DL_{CO} (Eq. 1).
2. Pregnancy usually reduces the DL_{CO} by approximately 15%, but the mechanism is not fully understood.
3. With an isolated, unexplained reduction in DL_{CO} (with normal results on spirometry and normal lung volumes), pulmonary vascular disease, such as primary pulmonary

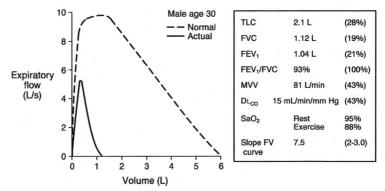

TLC	2.1 L	(28%)
FVC	1.12 L	(19%)
FEV₁	1.04 L	(21%)
FEV₁/FVC	93%	(100%)
MVV	81 L/min	(43%)
DL_CO	15 mL/min/mm Hg	(43%)
SaO₂	Rest	95%
	Exercise	88%
Slope FV curve	7.5	(2-3.0)

FIG. 4-2. Case of severe restrictive disease. Total lung capacity (TLC) is markedly reduced, the ratio of forced expiratory volume in 1 second to forced vital capacity (FEV_1/FVC) is normal, the carbon monoxide diffusing capacity of the lung (DL_{CO}) is reduced, and the oxygen saturation (SaO_2) is decreased with exercise. The maximal voluntary ventilation (MVV) is not as severely reduced as the FEV_1; thus, the calculation of $FEV_1 \times 40$ does not work in this situation. The steep slope of the flow-volume (FV) curve and the reduced DL_{CO} suggest a pulmonary parenchymal cause of the severe restriction. The diagnosis in this case was idiopathic pulmonary fibrosis. Numbers in parentheses are percent of predicted, except for slope FV curve, in which numbers are a range.

hypertension, recurrent pulmonary emboli, or obliterative vasculopathy, should be considered.

Figures 4-2 through 4-4 present cases in which knowledge of the DL_{CO} is very useful.

4F. OTHER CONSIDERATIONS

The test for DL_{CO} is very sensitive. We have found transient decreases of 3 to 5 mL/min per mm Hg with mild respiratory infections in normal subjects. It is a useful test for following the course of patients with idiopathic pulmonary fibrosis or sarcoidosis and for evaluating therapeutic interventions. The test has also been used to follow the extent of intra-alveolar hemorrhage in conditions such as Goodpasture's syndrome.

One might expect changes in the resting DL_{CO} to be closely correlated with the arterial oxygen tension (PaO_2). However, this is not always so. For example, with lung resection DL_{CO} is reduced,

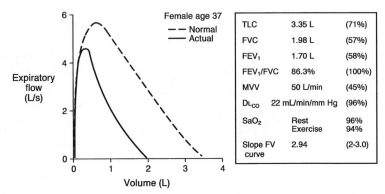

	Female age 37		
	— — Normal		
	—— Actual		
TLC	3.35 L	(71%)	
FVC	1.98 L	(57%)	
FEV$_1$	1.70 L	(58%)	
FEV$_1$/FVC	86.3%	(100%)	
MVV	50 L/min	(45%)	
D$_{LCO}$	22 mL/min/mm Hg	(96%)	
SaO$_2$	Rest	96%	
	Exercise	94%	
Slope FV curve	2.94	(2-3.0)	

FIG. 4-3.   As with Figure 4-2, this pattern is consistent with a restrictive process (reduced TLC, FVC, and FEV$_1$, and a normal FEV$_1$/FVC ratio). However, it differs from the case in Figure 4-2 in that the D$_{LCO}$ is normal, as is the slope of the FV curve. The MVV is also low. Further testing revealed a severe reduction in respiratory muscle strength (see Chapter 9), consistent with the diagnosis of amyotrophic lateral sclerosis. (Abbreviations are defined in the legend to Fig. 4-2.)

but the Pao$_2$ is generally normal. However, a low resting D$_{LCO}$ often correlates with a decrease in Pao$_2$ during exercise.

PEARL: A D$_{LCO}$ of less than 50% of predicted suggests a pulmonary vascular or parenchymal disorder. In a patient with a normal chest radiograph and no evidence of airway obstruction, this should lead to

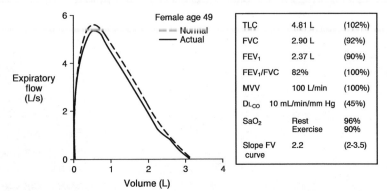

	Female age 49		
	— — Normal		
	—— Actual		
TLC	4.81 L	(102%)	
FVC	2.90 L	(92%)	
FEV$_1$	2.37 L	(90%)	
FEV$_1$/FVC	82%	(100%)	
MVV	100 L/min	(100%)	
D$_{LCO}$	10 mL/min/mm Hg	(45%)	
SaO$_2$	Rest	96%	
	Exercise	90%	
Slope FV curve	2.2	(2-3.5)	

FIG. 4-4.   In this case there is no apparent ventilatory limitation, the area under the FV curve being normal. All test values are normal except for the striking reduction in the D$_{LCO}$ and the desaturation with exercise. Primary pulmonary hypertension was diagnosed. (Abbreviations are defined in the legend to Fig. 4-2.)

further investigation, such as high-resolution computed tomography, to look for interstitial changes or a pulmonary vascular study, such as echocardiography, to measure pulmonary artery pressure.

REFERENCES

1. American Thoracic Society. Single-breath carbon monoxide diffusing capacity (transfer factor): recommendations for a standard technique—1995 update. *Am J Respir Crit Care Med* 152:2185–2198, 1995.
2. Crapo RO, Jensen RL, Wanger JS. Single-breath carbon monoxide diffusing capacity. *Clin Chest Med* 22:637–649, 2001.

5

Bronchodilators and Bronchial Challenge Testing

When a patient undergoes pulmonary function tests for the first time, it is almost always worthwhile to have spirometry performed before and after the administration of an inhaled bronchodilator.

5A. REASONS FOR BRONCHODILATOR TESTING

Administering a β_2 agonist is rarely contraindicated. Ipratropium bromide can be used if the β_2 agonist is contraindicated. The major values of bronchodilator testing are as follows:

1. If the patient shows a positive response (see below), one is inclined to treat more aggressively with bronchodilators and possibly with inhaled corticosteroids. The improvement can be shown to the patient, and compliance is thus often improved. However, even if no measurable improvement occurs, a therapeutic trial (2 wk) of an inhaled bronchodilator in patients with obstructive disease may provide symptomatic and objective improvement.
2. Patients with chronic obstructive pulmonary disease (COPD) who acutely show a heightened response to a bronchodilator have been found to have an accelerated decrease in pulmonary function over time. In such cases, aggressive therapy of the COPD seems warranted.

> **PEARL:** Some pulmonologists believe that a positive response to a bronchodilator in COPD warrants a trial of corticosteroid therapy, preferably by inhaled aerosol. Although inhaled corticosteroids are commonly used in COPD, especially for patients who improve with a bronchodilator, four recent randomized clinical trials failed to show benefit, except in secondary analyses that showed some relief of symptoms of severe COPD and slightly less frequent exacerbations [1].

3. Possibly the most important result is the detection of unsuspected asthma in a subject with low-normal results on spirometry.

5B. ADMINISTRATION OF BRONCHODILATOR

The agent can be administered either by a nebulizer unit or by use of a metered-dose inhaler. The technique for the inhaler is described in Figure 5-1.

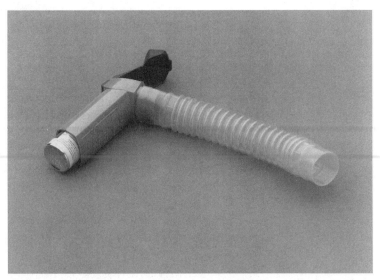

FIG. 5-1. Technique for use of metered-dose inhaler. An inexpensive spacer of 5 to 6 in. is cut from disposable ventilator tubing. The patient is told to exhale toward residual volume, place the tubing in the mouth with lips around the tubing, and begin a slow, deep inspiration. The metered-dose inhaler is activated once at the start of inspiration, which continues to total lung capacity. The patient holds his or her breath for 6 to 10 seconds and then quietly exhales. After a few normal breaths, the procedure is repeated.

Ideally, the patient should not have used a bronchodilator before testing. Abstinence of 6 hours from the inhaled β_2 agonists and anticholinergics and 12 hours from long-acting β_2 agonists, salmeterol or formoterol, and methylxanthines is recommended. The technician should always record whether and when the medications were last taken. Use of corticosteroids need not be discontinued.

5C. INTERPRETATION OF RESPONSE

The American Thoracic Society defines a significant bronchodilator response as one in which the forced expiratory volume in 1 second (FEV_1) or the forced vital capacity (FVC) increases by *both* 12% and 200 mL.

> **PEARL:** To evaluate whether the increase in FVC is merely the result of a prolonged effort, overlay the control and postdilator curves so that the starting volumes are the same, as in Figure 5-2B. If there is a slight increase in flow, then the increase in FVC is not due to prolonged effort alone.

The forced expiratory flow rate over the middle 50% of the FVC (FEF_{25-75}) is a useful measure of airway obstruction. It is *not* a reliable indicator of an acute change in maximal expiratory flow, however, because of the way it is affected by changes in the FVC, as shown in Figure 5-2. Typical normal and abnormal responses to inhaled bronchodilator are shown in Figure 5-3.

5D. EFFECT OF EFFORT ON INTERPRETATION

In routine spirometry, changing effort can have a misleading effect on the FEV_1 and flow-volume curve. In Figure 5-4 the same subject has made two consecutive acceptable FVC efforts. During one (curve a) the subject made a maximal effort with a high peak flow and sustained maximal effort throughout the breath. However, in another effort (curve b), the subject *initially* exhaled with slightly less than maximal force for less than a second and thereafter applied the same maximal effort as in curve a. The peak expiratory flow was slightly lower on curve b, but the flow on curve b exceeds

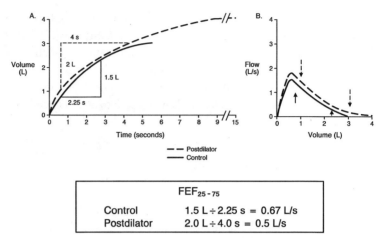

	FEF$_{25-75}$
Control	1.5 L ÷ 2.25 s = 0.67 L/s
Postdilator	2.0 L ÷ 4.0 s = 0.5 L/s

FIG. 5-2.   By definition, the FEF$_{25-75}$ (forced expiratory flow rate) is measured over the middle 50% of the vital capacity (**A**). The spirograms and flow-volume curves show an increase in both flow and volume after use of a bronchodilator. Yet the control FEF$_{25-75}$ (0.67 L/s) is higher than the postdilator value (0.5 L/s). The reason for this apparent paradox can be appreciated from the FV curves (**B**). The *solid arrows* indicate the volume range over which the control FEF$_{25-75}$ is calculated. The *dashed arrows* show the volume range over which the postdilator FEF$_{25-75}$ is calculated. The flows are lower at the end of the 25 to 75% volume range on the postdilator curve than those on the control curve. More time is spent at the low flows, which, in turn, causes the postdilator FEF$_{25-75}$ to be lower than the control value. **Recommendation:** Do not use the FEF$_{25-75}$ to evaluate bronchodilator response. Instead use the forced expiratory volume in 1 second and *always* look at the curves.

that on curve a at lower volumes. In this situation, the slightly less forceful effort can produce an FEV$_1$ that may be 15% higher than the maximal effort. This result could be interpreted as a significant bronchodilator effect. Clearly, the subject's lungs and airways have not changed, however. The increase of FEV$_1$ with less effort shown on curve b can be considered an artifact resulting from the slight difference in initial effort.

There is a physiologic explanation for this apparent paradox, and the interested reader is referred to Krowka and associates [2], but it is sufficient that one be alert to this potentially confusing occurrence. The best way to avoid this problem is to require that all flow-volume curves have sharp peak flows, as in curve a on Figure 5-4, especially when two efforts are compared. Short of that, the peak flows should be very nearly identical. The principle also applies to bronchial challenge testing (see below). This

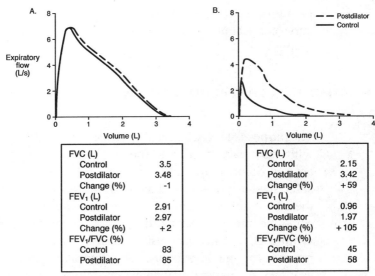

FVC (L)	
Control	3.5
Postdilator	3.48
Change (%)	-1
FEV₁ (L)	
Control	2.91
Postdilator	2.97
Change (%)	+2
FEV₁/FVC (%)	
Control	83
Postdilator	85

FVC (L)	
Control	2.15
Postdilator	3.42
Change (%)	+59
FEV₁ (L)	
Control	0.96
Postdilator	1.97
Change (%)	+105
FEV₁/FVC (%)	
Control	45
Postdilator	58

FIG. 5-3. Responses to inhaled bronchodilator. **A.** Normal response with −1% change in the forced vital capacity (FVC) and +2% change in the forced expiratory volume in 1 second (FEV₁). **B.** Positive response with a 59% increase in the FVC and a 105% increase in the FEV₁. The FEV₁/FVC ratio is relatively insensitive to this change and therefore should not be used to evaluate bronchodilator response.

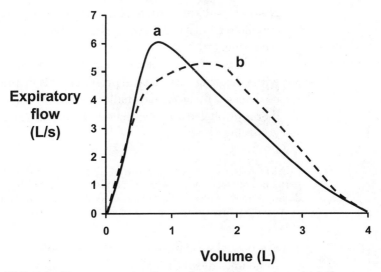

FIG. 5-4. Two consecutive flow-volume curves during which the subject exerted maximal effort (curve a) and then slightly submaximal effort (curve b). Note the slightly lower and delayed peak flow but higher flows over the lower volumes of curve b.

paradoxical behavior can easily be identified from flow-volume curves; it is almost impossible to recognize it from volume-time graphs.

5E. INDICATIONS FOR BRONCHIAL CHALLENGE TESTING

The purpose of bronchial challenge testing is to detect the patient with hyperreactive airways. The classic example of hyperreactive airways occurs in the patient with bronchial asthma. Various insults, such as pollens, cold air, exercise, smoke, and dust, cause the smooth airway muscles to constrict and the mucosa to become inflamed. Wheezing, dyspnea, and cough are the classic symptoms, and the diagnosis is clear-cut. Not all patients with hyperreactive airways fit this classic clinical picture, however. For example, the patient may complain only of cough. In such patients, bronchial challenge testing can be extremely useful. Failure to recognize the existence of patients who do not have classic symptoms has contributed to the underutilization of bronchial challenge. The most common indications for this procedure are the following:

1. Normal results of spirometry and a normal response to bronchodilators but a history suggesting asthma with occasional wheezing.
2. Chronic cough that is often worse at night but not associated with wheezing. Asthma can present in this manner and can be detected by bronchial challenge testing. The response to therapy (inhaled bronchodilators and corticosteroids) can be gratifying.

PEARL: Asthma is often a nocturnal disease. According to some experts, if a subject does not have symptoms at night, then the subject does not have asthma. This principle does not necessarily apply, however, to the patient with exercise- or cold-air–induced asthma.

3. Episodic chest tightness often accompanied by cough and sometimes dyspnea. This is a common presentation of non-wheezing hyperreactive airways, a variant of asthma.
4. Occult asthma, which should always be in the differential diagnosis of unexplained dyspnea.

5. Recurrent episodes of chest colds, bronchitis, or recurrent pneumonia with infiltrates that do not occur in the same lung regions. This can occur with occult asthma. Detecting and treating hyperreactive airways in this situation can lead to substantial clinical improvement.

6. Unexplained decrease in exercise tolerance, not perceived as dyspnea and often occurring in cold air. Exercise and cold air are well-known triggers of asthma.

Bronchial challenge testing is often positive in patients with allergic rhinitis, sarcoidosis (50% of cases), COPD, and cystic fibrosis.

> **PEARL:** It is often wise to follow up a borderline or mildly positive bronchodilator response with a methacholine challenge. A 52-year-old woman had a history of cough and shortness of breath. Initial tests were normal in this nonsmoker, and there was only a 9% increase in the FEV_1 after a bronchodilator. However, a methacholine challenge resulted in a 38% decrease in FEV_1 associated with cough and dyspnea, both of which were reversed by a bronchodilator. The patient clearly had asthma.

5F. PROCEDURE FOR BRONCHIAL CHALLENGE TESTING

The most commonly used agent for bronchoprovocation is inhaled methacholine, a cholinergic drug that stimulates muscarinic receptors and causes contraction of smooth muscle in the airway. The degree to which the smooth muscle contracts depends on its reactivity and is reflected in the magnitude of decrease in expiratory flow, usually quantified by measuring the FEV_1.

On exposure to an allergen, a person with asthma may experience an initial (within a few minutes) decrease in expiratory flow, which is called the "immediate" response. This is what is measured in bronchial challenge testing. It can be blocked by bronchodilators and cromolyn sodium. In asthma, there may also be a "late" or "delayed" response, which usually occurs 4 to 12 hours after exposure; it reflects the airway inflammatory response. This response can be blocked by corticosteroids or cromolyn sodium and is not elicited by methacholine. Allergens such as pollens may elicit either response or both the "early" and "late" responses. Although methacholine provokes only the early phase of the classic asthmatic hyperreactive airway response, it nevertheless is an

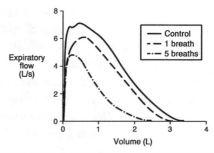

	Control	1 breath	5 breaths
FVC (L)	3.49	3.1	2.47
FEV₁ (L)	2.86	2.54	1.82
FEV₁ (% decrease)		11	36
FEV₁/FVC (%)	82	82	74

FIG. 5-5.   Results of bronchial challenge testing in a 43-year-old woman who had a 3-year history of persistent cough, often at night. She denied wheezing but had mild dyspnea on exertion. One breath of methacholine produced a parallel shift in the FV curve, no change in the ratio of forced expiratory volume in 1 second to forced vital capacity (FEV_1/FVC), a decrease of 11% in the FEV_1, and mild chest tightness. She was given four additional breaths of methacholine, and cough and chest tightness developed, but there was no audible wheezing. This is a positive test result with a 36% decrease in the FEV_1. Note that at five breaths, the FV curve shows scooping and is no longer parallel with the control curve. The curve after one breath demonstrates that mild bronchoconstriction may produce only a mild decrease in FEV_1 and no change in the FEV_1/FVC ratio (see section 3E, page 35 and Fig. 3-8A, page 38). Further constriction (curve after five breaths) leads to a FV curve that is classic for obstruction, with scooping, a low FEV_1, and a decreased FEV_1/FVC ratio.

excellent predictor of the presence of asthma. Thus, a positive result on methacholine challenge testing is predictive of asthma attacks provoked by, for example, cold air, exercise, pollens, or infection. An example of a positive methacholine challenge study is illustrated in Figure 5-5.

Several protocols have been developed for bronchial challenge testing [3]. Clinically, the goal is to determine whether the patient has asthma. For this purpose, we favor a simple screening procedure such as described by Parker and associates [4] in 1965. The procedure is as follows:

1. Five milliliters of a 25 mg/mL solution of methacholine chloride in normal saline is freshly prepared, and 2 to 3 mL is

placed in a standard nebulizer. It is not advisable to subject a patient to bronchial challenge if the baseline FEV_1 is less than 65% of predicted. If the FEV_1 is between 65 and 75% of predicted, the test is done with caution. If very hyperreactive airways are suspected, a concentration of 5 mg/mL or lower is used rather than 25 mg/mL. The low concentration is used in children, who often show a very severe response.

2. Baseline spirometry is performed to obtain a reproducible FEV_1. The subject then inhales a deep breath of methacholine, holds the breath for 5 to 10 seconds, and then breathes quietly.

3. Spirometry is repeated in 1 minute to obtain two reproducible measurements of FEV_1. If the FEV_1 has decreased by 20%, the result is positive. If the FEV_1 has decreased less than 15%, four more breaths of methacholine are inhaled. If the decrease is between 15 and 19%, only two more breaths are inhaled.

4. Spirometry is repeated in 1 minute.

A response is *positive* if the FEV_1 decreases by 20% or more of control. In this case, a β_2 agonist is administered to reverse the effect of the methacholine.

Technicians should always note whether the methacholine causes symptoms, such as chest tightness, substernal burning, cough, or wheezing. If the patient's symptoms are reproduced but the decrease in FEV_1 is less than but near to 20% (15–19%), we are inclined to consider that a borderline positive result.

Clinicians need to always be alert to the confounding effect of effort dependence on the FEV_1 (see page 53 and Fig. 5-4). For example, a control effort that is less than maximal may yield a value of FEV_1 that is falsely high compared with the value on a truly maximal effort after the inhalation of methacholine. A decrease in FEV_1 in this situation could be due to varying effort and *not* hyperreactive airways.

There are, of course, modifications to this approach that can be considered. For example, in a patient who becomes dyspneic or has chest tightness when cross-country skiing, cold air may be the cause. Baseline spirometry needs to be performed. Then the patient should walk or jog outside to reproduce the symptoms, and retest is done immediately after the patient comes inside. The question of whether workplace exposure is causing symptoms can similarly be evaluated by testing before and immediately after work.

Also, the following points need to be kept in mind:

1. Normal subjects may show a transient (for several months) increase in bronchial reactivity after viral respiratory infections, but they do not necessarily have asthma. This phenomenon is called the postviral airway hyperresponsiveness syndrome, and generally it responds well to inhaled bronchodilator and corticosteroid therapy.

2. In some persons with asthma, deep inspirations, such as occur with FVC maneuvers, can cause bronchoconstriction. This can lead to a progressive decrease in the FVC and FEV_1 on repeated efforts during routine testing.

3. Patients with hyperreactive airways (that is, a positive result on methacholine challenge) may have an exacerbation of asthma or a severe asthma attack if given a β-adrenergic blocking agent. For example, this situation has been reported with use of eyedrops for the treatment of glaucoma, in which the eyedrops contain a β-adrenergic antagonist.

4. Many patients with COPD or chronic bronchitis have an increase in bronchial reactivity. Their results on methacholine challenge will usually be between those of normal subjects and persons with asthma. The clinical history is usually sufficiently different in the two groups to permit distinction; however, there can be considerable overlap, leading to confusion in diagnosis and treatment.

5. Airway reactivity may vary over time. Airway responsiveness in asthma improves with long-term inhaled corticosteroid therapy. The degree of responsiveness correlates with the degree of airway narrowing because narrowed airways need to constrict only slightly to increase resistance markedly.

REFERENCES

1. The Lung Health Study Research Group. Effect of inhaled triamcinolone on the decline in pulmonary function in chronic obstructive pulmonary disease. *N Engl J Med* 343:1902–1909, 2000.

2. Krowka MJ, Enright PL, Rodarte JR, Hyatt RE. Effect of effort on measurement of forced expiratory volume in one second. *Am Rev Respir Dis* 136:829–833, 1987.
3. Crapo RO, Casaburi R, Coates AL, et al. Guidelines for methacholine and exercise challenge testing—1999. *Am J Respir Crit Care Med* 161:309–329, 2000.
4. Parker CD, Bilbo RE, Reed CE. Methacholine aerosol as test for bronchial asthma. *Arch Intern Med* 115:452–458, 1965.

6

Arterial Blood Gases

Arterial blood gas analysis is performed to answer various clinical questions: Is gas exchange normal? Is there carbon dioxide retention in the patient with chronic obstructive pulmonary disease (COPD), severe asthma, or severe restrictive disease? Is there hypoxemia (low oxygen saturation)? Does the saturation decrease with exercise? What is the acid-base status?

Several important aspects need to be considered for obtaining and handling arterial blood specimens. The laboratory must always indicate on the report form whether the patient was breathing room air or an increased oxygen concentration. As stated in section 3B (page 29), the arterial oxygen tension may be lower in the supine position than the upright posture. Therefore, the posture of the patient should be noted. The patient should be neither hyperventilating nor holding his or her breath. The specimen should not contain any air bubbles, and it should be quickly iced and promptly analyzed. Similar precautions apply to analysis of the pH of pleural fluid when empyema is a possibility.

6A. ARTERIAL OXYGEN TENSION

There are four major steps in the transfer of oxygen from inhaled air to the tissues:

1. *Ventilation* of the alveoli must be adequate.
2. Within the lung, the inhaled air must come in contact with venous blood; that is, there must be adequate *matching of ventilation ($\dot{V}$) to perfusion ($\dot{Q}$)*.
3. There must be *diffusion* of the oxygen through the alveolar wall into the hemoglobin in the red cells (see Chapter 4).

4. Oxygenated hemoglobin must then be transported by the cardiovascular system to the tissues.

The first two steps are discussed in this chapter. Transport or so-called internal respiration deals with the oxygen content of blood, the cardiac output, and the distribution of blood flow to the organs, and this topic is outside the province of this book.

The tension of oxygen in the arterial blood (Pao_2) reflects the adequacy of the transfer of oxygen from ambient air to blood. In normal young adults, the Pao_2 values at sea level range from 85 to 100 mm Hg. The values decrease slightly with age, to about 80 mm Hg at age 70. *Hypoxemia* exists when the Pao_2 is less than these values. The oxygen dissociation curve is useful in the consideration of hypoxemia. Figure 6-1 shows the average values for the oxygen tension of mixed venous blood (v $\sim$ $P\bar{v}o_2$ = 40 mm Hg, saturation 75%) and arterial blood (a $\sim$ Pao_2 = 100 mm Hg, saturation 96%). The curve is very steep at and below the venous point where small changes in oxygen tension produce dramatic change in the oxygen content of blood, and hence the saturation. Conversely, at oxygen tensions of more than 60 to 70 mm Hg, large changes in tension have a relatively small effect on saturation. Hence, very

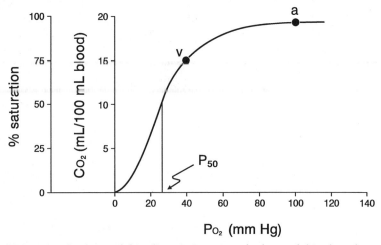

FIG. 6-1. Oxyhemoglobin dissociation curve for hemoglobin that plots oxygen saturation against the partial pressure of oxygen (Po_2) and also the oxygen content (Co_2). P_{50} is the partial pressure of oxygen that results in a 50% saturation of hemoglobin. a, arterial blood; v, mixed venous blood. (From AE Taylor, K Rehder, RE Hyatt, et al [eds]. *Clinical Respiratory Physiology*. Philadelphia: Saunders, 1989. By permission of publisher.)

little additional oxygen can normally be added to the blood by using very high inspired oxygen tensions. Cyanosis is not easily appreciated until the saturation has decreased to less than 75%.

The four common causes of hypoxemia occurring with a *normal* inspired oxygen tension are hypoventilation, ventilation-perfusion ($\dot{V}/\dot{Q}$) mismatch, shunt, and impaired diffusion.

Hypoventilation

This refers specifically to *alveolar* hypoventilation. There are two important, distinguishing features of alveolar hypoventilation. One feature is that arterial carbon dioxide tension ($Paco_2$) is always increased. The following simple equation defines the relationship between $Paco_2$ and alveolar ventilation ($\dot{V}A$) and carbon dioxide production by the body ($\dot{V}co_2$) ("k" is a constant):

$$Paco_2 = k \times \frac{\dot{V}co_2}{\dot{V}A} \qquad \text{(Eq. 1)}$$

Assume $\dot{V}co_2$ stays constant. When ($\dot{V}A$) decreases, $Paco_2$ must increase. Similarly, an increase in $\dot{V}co_2$ can increase $Paco_2$.

A way to think of alveolar ventilation is as follows. When a subject inhales a tidal volume breath (designated VT), a certain amount of that breath does not reach the gas-exchanging alveoli. A portion stays in the upper airway, trachea, and bronchi, and a portion may go to alveoli with no perfusion (especially in disease), so that gas exchange does not occur in either case. This fraction of the inhaled VT is referred to as the dead space volume (VD). The VD is small in normal conditions but increased in diseases such as emphysema and chronic bronchitis. If total ventilation ($\dot{V}E$) is defined as the ventilation measured at the mouth, then

$$\dot{V}A = \dot{V}E - \dot{V}E \left(\frac{VD}{VT}\right) \qquad \text{(Eq. 2)}$$

That is, alveolar ventilation is the total ventilation minus the amount ventilating the dead space. Thus, $\dot{V}A$ in Equation 1 is decreased by a decrease in $\dot{V}E$ or by an increase in VD/VT.

The second feature is that the hypoxemia due to alveolar hypoventilation can always be corrected by increasing the inspired oxygen concentration. An increase of approximately 1 mm Hg in inspired oxygen tension produces a 1-mm Hg increase in arterial oxygen tension. Inspired oxygen can be increased several hundred millimeters of mercury, and the hypoxemia is easily corrected. Some of the more common causes of hypoventilation are listed in Table 6-1; all reflect abnormalities in the function of the respiratory pump.

Hypoventilation can be identified as a cause of hypoxia with use of the alveolar air equation:

$$P_{AO_2} = (P_{atm} - P_{H_2O})\, F_{IO_2} - \left(\frac{P_{ACO_2}}{RQ}\right) \qquad \text{(Eq. 3)}$$

where P_{AO_2} is the partial pressure of oxygen in the alveoli, P_{atm} is atmospheric pressure, P_{H_2O} is the partial pressure of water (47 mm Hg at body temperature), F_{IO_2} is the fraction of inspired oxygen, P_{ACO_2} is the partial pressure of carbon dioxide in the alveoli, and RQ is respiratory quotient (usually 0.7-0.8 with a normal diet). $P_{AO_2} - P_{aO_2}$ is usually called the A-a gradient or, $(A-a)\, D_{O_2}$. It is typically less than 10 in a young person and less than 20 in an older person. If it is normal, hypoxia is due to hypoventilation or a low F_{IO_2}. If it is high, hypoxia may be due to $\dot{V}/\dot{Q}$ mismatch, shunt, or diffusion impairment.

Ventilation-Perfusion Mismatch

Instead of the normal situation in which nearly equal volumes of air and venous blood go to all alveoli, a disparity (mismatch) may develop. Increased blood flow ($\dot{Q}$) may go to alveoli whose ventilation ($\dot{V}$) is reduced. Conversely, increased ventilation may go to areas with reduced blood flow. The result in either case is impaired gas exchange, often of a significant degree. In the ultimate hypothetical mismatch, all the blood goes to one lung and all the ventilation to the other, a situation incompatible with life. In the real-life situation, hypoxemia due to $\dot{V}/\dot{Q}$ mismatch can be improved and usually corrected by increased inspired oxygen concentrations unless the mismatch is extreme.

$\dot{V}/\dot{Q}$ mismatch is the most common cause of hypoxemia encountered in clinical practice. It explains the hypoxemia in chronic bronchitis, emphysema, and asthma. It also explains much of the hypoxemia in interstitial lung disease and pulmonary edema.

Estimating the degree and type of mismatch is complex and beyond the scope of this book. Suffice it to say, an *increase* in the $(A-a)D_{O_2}$ most often suggests the existence of lung regions with a low $\dot{V}/\dot{Q}$ ratio, due to perfusion exceeding ventilation. The so-called physiologic dead space (VD) can also be estimated; an increase implies the existence of lung regions with a high $\dot{V}/\dot{Q}$ ratio due to a relative increase in ventilation. To pursue this interesting subject further, the reader should consult a standard text of respiratory physiology.

Right-to-Left Shunt

In this situation, a quantity of venous blood totally bypasses the alveoli. The shunt may be extrapulmonary, as in atrial septal defect or tetralogy of Fallot, or it may occur within the lung, such as with arteriovenous fistulae in hereditary hemorrhagic telangiectasia (the Osler-Weber-Rendu syndrome). Blood flow through a region of total pneumonic consolidation or atelectasis also constitutes a right-to-left shunt. In shunt, the hypoxemia *cannot* be abolished by breathing 100% oxygen.

Impaired Diffusion

Diffusion is discussed in detail in Chapter 4. As mentioned before, $\dot{V}/\dot{Q}$ mismatch may contribute to the reduction in the diffusing capacity that is measured in the laboratory. Breathing a high-oxygen concentration can usually correct the hypoxemia caused by the diffusion impairment.

Mixed Causes

There are also mixed causes of hypoxemia. The patient with COPD and pneumonia has both $\dot{V}/\dot{Q}$ mismatch and right-to-left shunting. The patient with pulmonary fibrosis has both a diffusion defect and $\dot{V}/\dot{Q}$ mismatch.

6B. ARTERIAL CARBON DIOXIDE TENSION

The normal values for Pa_{CO_2} range from 35 to 45 mm Hg and, unlike Pa_{O_2}, are not affected by age. Figure 6-2 contrasts the dissociation curve of carbon dioxide with that of oxygen. The carbon dioxide curve does not have a plateau. Thus, the carbon dioxide content of blood is strongly dependent on Pa_{CO_2}, which in turn is exquisitely sensitive to the level of alveolar ventilation (Eq. 1).

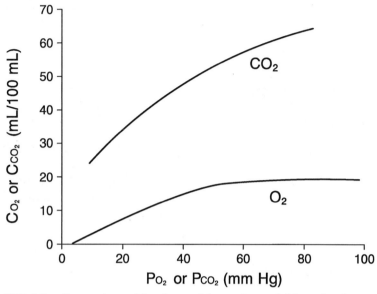

FIG. 6-2. Comparison of the shape of the oxyhemoglobin and carbon dioxide dissociation curves. The slope of the carbon dioxide dissociation curve is about three times steeper than that of the oxyhemoglobin dissociation curve. C_{CO_2} is the carbon dioxide content of blood, C_{O_2} is the oxygen content of blood, and P_{CO_2} and P_{O_2} are the partial pressures of carbon dioxide and oxygen in blood, respectively. (Modified from JB West [ed]. *Respiratory Physiology—The Essentials* [3rd ed]. Baltimore: Williams & Wilkins, 1985. By permission of publisher.)

Hypercapnia (that is, carbon dioxide retention with increased P_{aCO_2}) can result from either of two mechanisms. The first mechanism, hypoventilation (Table 6-1), is more readily understood. Section 6A explains that P_{aCO_2} is inversely proportional to alveolar ventilation (Eq. 1). When alveolar ventilation decreases, P_{aCO_2} increases.

The second mechanism is that severe $\dot{V}/\dot{Q}$ mismatch can also lead to carbon dioxide retention. When P_{aO_2} decreases as a result of $\dot{V}/\dot{Q}$ mismatch, as discussed previously, P_{aCO_2} increases. This commonly occurs in COPD. However, in some patients ventilation increases to maintain a normal P_{aCO_2}. P_{aO_2} also improves some. These are the so-called pink puffers. In other patients with COPD, the P_{aCO_2} increases and the P_{aO_2} decreases as a result of $\dot{V}/\dot{Q}$ mismatch. These are the classic "blue bloaters," the cyanotic hypoventilators. Of course, many patients with COPD have a course between these two extremes.

TABLE 6-1. Some causes of alveolar hypoventilation

Central nervous system depression caused by drugs, anesthesia,
    hypothyroidism
Disorders of the medullary respiratory center caused by trauma,
    hemorrhage, encephalitis, stroke, tumor
Disorders of respiratory control such as sleep apnea and the obesity
    hypoventilation syndrome
Chest trauma with flail chest, kyphoscoliosis, thoracoplasty
Neuromuscular disease affecting the efferent nerves (such as
    poliomyelitis, Guillain-Barré syndrome, and amyotrophic lateral
    sclerosis); the neuromuscular junction (such as myasthenia gravis); or
    the respiratory muscles (such as muscular dystrophy, acid maltase
    deficiency, and other myopathies)

6C. ARTERIAL pH

pH is the negative log of the hydrogen ion concentration. This means that in acidosis (low pH) there is an increase in H^+ ions. The converse holds for alkalosis, with its decrease in H^+ ions and increased pH.

The acid-base status of the blood is classically analyzed in terms of the Henderson-Hasselbalch equation for the bicarbonate buffer system, which highlights the importance of the arterial partial pressure of carbon dioxide (P_{CO_2}).

$$pH = pK + \log \frac{[HCO_3^-]}{0.03 \, P_{CO_2}} \qquad \text{(Eq. 2)}$$

The pK is a constant related to the dissociation of carbonic acid. Note that with constant bicarbonate, increases in the P_{CO_2} lower the pH. Conversely, lowering the P_{CO_2} by increasing ventilation produces alkalosis (increased pH).

Respiratory alterations in acid-base status are related to elimination of carbon dioxide. Metabolic abnormalities, however, entail either a gain or a loss of fixed acid or bicarbonate in the extracellular fluid. Metabolic alterations in acid-base balance are rapidly compensated for by alternating the amount of carbon dioxide eliminated by ventilation. This is followed by the slower elimination by the kidneys of excess acid or base.

The Davenport pH-[HCO_3^-] diagram shown in Figure 6-3 is a useful way of looking at the body's response to acid-base alterations. It is a graphic representation of the Henderson-Hasselbalch

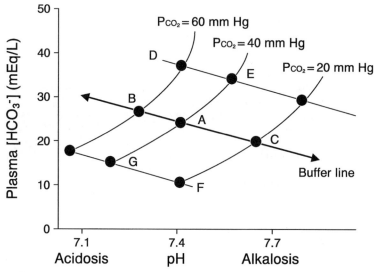

FIG. 6-3. Davenport diagram showing [HCO$_3^-$] as a function of pH and partial pressure of carbon dioxide (Pco$_2$). (From AE Taylor, K Rehder, RE Hyatt, et al [eds]. *Clinical Respiratory Physiology.* Philadelphia: Saunders, 1989. By permission of publisher.)

equation. Shown are three different buffer lines (slanting down and to the right) defining the [HCO$_3^-$] and pH responses resulting from adding metabolic acid or base to plasma. Also shown are three isopleths (slanting up and to the right) relating pH to [HCO$_3^-$] for three levels of Pco$_2$. Point A indicates the normal situation: pH = 7.4, [HCO$_3^-$] = 24 mEq/L, and Pco$_2$ = 40 mm Hg.

Compensatory Mechanisms

1. Respiratory acidosis: Point B in Figure 6-3 shows the result of acute hypoventilation; Pco$_2$ increases and pH decreases. The kidney seeks to compensate for the acidosis when hypoventilation becomes chronic, as in COPD, by conserving [HCO$_3^-$]. The result is that point B moves toward point D and pH returns toward normal.

2. Respiratory alkalosis: Point C shows what occurs with acute hyperventilation; Pco$_2$ decreases and pH increases. As hyperventilation persists, for example, during acclimatization to altitude, the kidneys excrete [HCO$_3^-$], and as predicted from Equation 2 the pH is normalized from C toward F.

3. Metabolic acidosis: Point G represents acidosis due to the accumulation of fixed acids with a lowering of plasma $[HCO_3^-]$. The respiratory system attempts to compensate by increasing ventilation, thus lowering Pco_2 and moving from G toward F. The classic example is the hyperpnea of diabetic acidosis.

4. Metabolic alkalosis: Loss of fixed acids, as with repeated vomiting, causes a shift from A to E. The respiratory response is a decrease in ventilation resulting in an increase in Pco_2 and movement from E toward D.

6D. AN ALTERNATIVE APPROACH TO ACID-BASE ANALYSIS

An alternative approach to the Davenport diagram is preferred by some and may be easier to use in the community hospital. Not all laboratories that perform arterial blood gas analysis have a co-oximeter to determine the bicarbonate level. The bicarbonate level can be calculated with the Henderson equation, in which $[H^+]$ is the hydrogen ion concentration:

$$[H^+] = 24 \times \frac{Pco_2}{[HCO_3^-]} \qquad \text{(Eq. 3)}$$

This can be rearranged to calculate the bicarbonate concentration:

$$[HCO_3^-] = 24 \times \frac{Pco_2}{[H^+]} \qquad \text{(Eq. 4)}$$

The hydrogen ion concentration (in mEq) can be calculated from the pH. Typical values are listed in Table 6-2. Intermediate values

TABLE 6-2. Relation of pH to hydrogen ion concentration

pH	$[H^+]$
7.50	32
7.40	40
7.30	50
7.22	60
7.15	71
7.10	79
7.05	89
7.00	100

can be calculated by interpolation. Once the bicarbonate, the pH, and the Pco_2 values are found, the acid-base status can be determined, and respiratory and metabolic causes of acidosis and alkalosis can be distinguished, as discussed in section 6C and Figure 6-3. A complete discussion of acid-base disturbances is beyond the scope of this book.

6E. ADDITIONAL CONSIDERATIONS

Many blood gas laboratories use a co-oximeter to measure total hemoglobin (Hb), hemoglobin saturation, carboxyhemoglobin (COHb), and methemoglobin (MetHb) and to calculate bicarbonate and arterial oxygen-carrying capacity (Cao_2). In the emergency room, measurement of COHb and MetHb is valuable for detecting carbon monoxide poisoning and toxicity from various medications that cause methemoglobinemia. In the intensive care unit, arterial blood gas values are checked frequently, and co-oximeter results often provide the first sign of blood loss in patients who have a high risk of gastrointestinal hemorrhage.

Mandated procedures and inspections under the Clinical Laboratories Improvement Act have improved quality control in arterial blood gas laboratories. Physicians should be aware of issues related to sample contamination and calibration of medical instrumentation. A useful rule is that the sum of the Pco_2 and Po_2 should not exceed roughly 150 mm Hg with the subject breathing room air. If the sum is more than this, the instrument's calibration should be checked.

6F. SOME POSSIBLE PROBLEMS

Case 1

The following blood gas results are from a 40-year-old patient who was sitting when the arterial blood was drawn:

$Pao_2 = 110$ mm Hg

$Paco_2 = 30$ mm Hg

pH $= 7.50$

Question: How should these results be interpreted, and what is the underlying problem?

Answer: The data indicate uncompensated acute respiratory alkalosis. The patient was frightened by the needle and hyperventilated as the blood was drawn.

Case 2

The patient is a small, 70-year-old woman with lobar pneumonia. The Pa_{O_2} value on admission was 50 mm Hg and saturation was 80%; she was given 40% inspired oxygen. Two hours later the patient looked somewhat better, but the Pa_{O_2} value was not improved. However, when the saturation was measured by pulse oximetry, it had increased to 92%.

Question: What might be the cause of the disparity between the blood gas and oximetry data? If the blood gas study was correct, intubation was indicated.

Answer: The technician was asked to draw another blood sample while saturation was monitored by pulse oximetry. As this was done, it was obvious that the patient held her breath during the needlestick and blood sampling and saturation decreased. Because of her small lung volumes, further reduced by pneumonia, her alveolar oxygen tension decreased drastically, leading to the low Pa_{O_2}. In a sample drawn when she did not hold her breath, the Pa_{O_2} was 80 mm Hg and the saturation was 92%.

Case 3

A 55-year-old man is being evaluated for weakness and chronic cough. He has had progressive difficulty swallowing for 6 months. His chest radiograph shows small lung volumes and bibasilar atelectasis with a superior segment infiltrate in the left lower lobe. Partial pressure of oxygen (P_{O_2}) is 45 mm Hg breathing room air, and P_{CO_2} is 62 mm Hg.

Question: What is the cause of his hypoxia?

Answer: Hypoventilation due to respiratory muscle weakness (see Chapter 9). The A-a gradient is nearly normal. Despite the radiographic abnormalities, his $\dot{V}/\dot{Q}$ matching is still good. He is hypoxic because of his hypercapnia.

7

Other Tests of Lung Mechanics: Resistance and Compliance

The tests described here are usually performed in fully equipped laboratories. In the outpatient setting, they add relatively little to the basic evaluations discussed in previous chapters (spirometry, lung volumes, diffusing capacity, and arterial blood gases). However, these tests might be encountered in either graduate training or in laboratory reports and therefore are considered briefly. Also, understanding these concepts is important in the management of patients requiring mechanical ventilation.

7A. RESISTANCE

Resistance is the pressure required to produce a flow of 1 L/s into or out of the lung. The units are centimeters of water per liter per second (cm $H_2O/L/s$). This general concept is illustrated in Figure 7-1, in which the pertinent driving pressure (ΔP) is the pressure difference between the ends of the tubes. The pressure required to produce a flow of 1 L/s in a large tube is less than that in a small tube. Hence, the resistance (R) of the small tube is much higher than that of the large tube.

In the lung, measurement of the resistance of the entire system is of interest. Figure 7-2 illustrates how this can be obtained. Flow at the mouth can be measured with a flowmeter. The pressure driving the flow can be measured in either of *two* ways. Pleural pressure (Ppl) can be measured from a small balloon-catheter unit placed

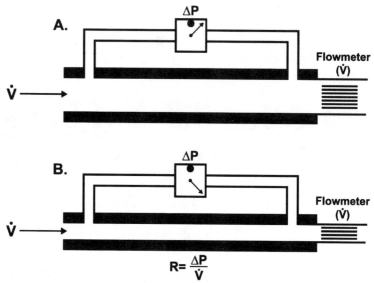

FIG. 7-1.   Measurement of resistance (R) through a large tube (**A**) and small tube (**B**). Flow (V̇) is measured by the flowmeter, and driving pressure (ΔP) is measured by a differential pressure transducer. To drive the same flow, the decrease in pressure is greater in tube **B**, and hence the resistance (R) of tube **B** is higher than that of tube **A**.

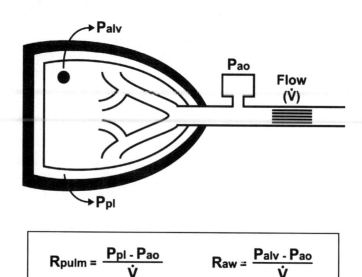

FIG. 7-2.   Model illustrating how pulmonary resistance (Rpulm) and airway resistance (Raw) are measured. An esophageal balloon is required to measure pleural pressure (Ppl). Palv, alveolar pressure; Pao, pressure at the mouth; V̇, flow.

in the lower third of the esophagus and attached to a pressure transducer. Pressure changes in the esophagus have been shown to reflect those in the pleural cavity. The difference between Ppl and Pao (the pressure at the mouth) is the driving pressure, which divided by flow ($\dot{V}$) is defined as the pulmonary resistance (Rpulm). Rpulm includes a small component due to the resistance of the lung tissue.

The other and much more common approach is to measure alveolar pressure (Palv) and relate this to Pao. Palv can be measured in a body plethysmograph and does not require swallowing an esophageal balloon. In this instance, the difference between Palv and Pao divided by flow is the airway resistance, Raw. Raw is slightly lower than Rpulm because of the absence of tissue resistance. Both Rpulm and Raw can be measured during either inspiration or expiration, or as an average of both. Figure 7-3 describes how Raw is measured.

Average resistance in normal adults is 1 to 3 cm $H_2O/L/s$. It is higher in the small lungs of children because the airways are

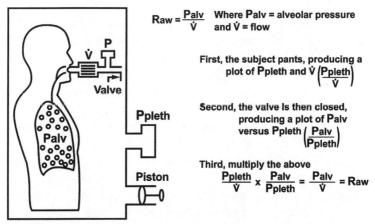

FIG. 7-3. The equipment used to measure lung volume by the body plethysmograph (see Fig. 3-6, page 34) has been modified by inserting a flowmeter between the patient's mouth and the pressure gauge and valve. The flowmeter measures airflow ($\dot{V}$). The subject is instructed to pant shallowly through the system with the valve open. This provides a measure of plethysmographic pressure as a function of flow, i.e., Ppleth/$\dot{V}$. With the subject still panting, the valve is closed. This provides a measure of alveolar pressure as a function of plethysmographic pressure, i.e., Palv/Ppleth. As shown, airway resistance (Raw) is obtained by multiplying these two ratios.

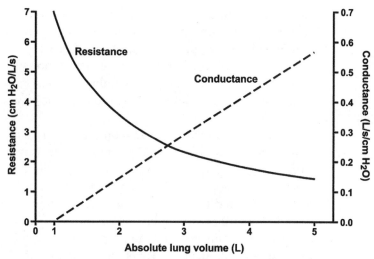

FIG. 7-4.   Resistance is a hyperbolic function of lung volume. When its reciprocal, conductance, is plotted, a straight line results. Note that the conductance line intersects the volume axis at 1 liter, which is the residual volume in this example. At the same time, resistance is becoming infinitely high.

smaller. Occasionally, the term conductance is used. *Conductance* is a term borrowed from the electrical engineering field and is the reciprocal of resistance, its units being liters per second per centimeter of water, L/s/cm H_2O. Thus, a high resistance means a low conductance—flow is not "conducted" well.

Resistance varies inversely with lung volume (Figure 7-4). At high lung volumes, the airways are wider and the resistance is lower. To standardize for this effect, resistance is typically measured during breathing at functional residual capacity.

Resistance is increased when the airways are narrowed. Narrowing may be due to bronchoconstriction of inflamed airways in asthma, mucus and thickened bronchi in chronic bronchitis, or floppy airways in emphysema.

There is a strong negative correlation between resistance and maximal expiratory flow. A high resistance is associated with decreased flows, evidenced by decreases in the forced expiratory volume in 1 second (FEV_1) and forced expiratory flow rate over the middle 50% of the forced vital capacity (FEF_{25-75}). There are, however, a few exceptions to this relationship. One is illustrated in Figure 7-5. This type of maximal expiratory flow-volume curve is occasionally seen in the elderly. Resistance in this case is normal,

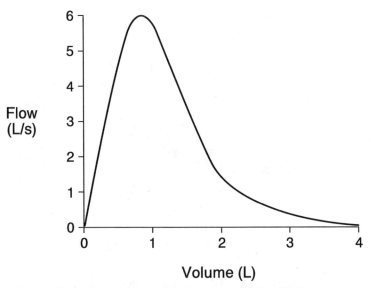

FIG. 7-5. Flow-volume curve showing normal flow at high lung volumes but abnormally low flows over the lower 50% of the vital capacity. In this case, resistance is often normal, but the forced expiratory flow rate over the middle 50% of the forced vital capacity is low.

but flow low in the vital capacity, such as the FEF$_{25-75}$, is decreased. The converse also can occur, namely, normal forced flows and an increased resistance.

> **PEARL:** A patient with a variable obstructing lesion in the extrathoracic trachea (see Fig. 2 7D, page 18) may have a significant increase in resistance but normal maximal expiratory flow. The increased resistance reflects the markedly decreased inspiratory flows caused by the high inspiratory resistance.

7B. PULMONARY COMPLIANCE

Compliance is a measure of the lung's elasticity. Compliance of the lungs (C$_L$) is defined as the change in lung volume resulting from a change of 1 cm H$_2$O in the elastic pressure of the lung. Figure 7-6 is similar to Figure 7-2, but a spirometer is added to measure volume (V). When the lung is not moving (that is, airflow is zero), the Ppl is negative (subatmospheric). The lungs are elastic and always tend to collapse. This is resisted by the chest wall, so the Ppl when volume is not changing reflects the static elastic pressure or recoil of the lung at that volume. If lung volume is increased by a known

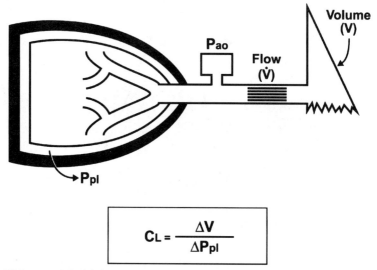

$$C_L = \frac{\Delta V}{\Delta P_{pl}}$$

FIG. 7-6. Model demonstrating the measurement of compliance. An esophageal balloon is required. C_L, compliance of the lungs; Pao, pressure at the mouth; Ppl, pleural pressure.

amount (ΔV) and volume is again held constant, the new Ppl is more negative (the recoil of the lung is greater). This ΔV divided by the difference in the two *static* Ppl values (ΔPpl) defines the lung compliance, $C_L = \Delta V / \Delta Ppl$ (L/cm H_2O). In addition, it is common practice to measure the elastic recoil pressure with the subject holding his or her breath at total lung capacity (TLC); this is termed the *PTLC* (recoil pressure at TLC). The measurement of lung compliance requires the introduction of an esophageal balloon (to measure Ppl).

Compliance measured when there is no airflow, as in the above discussion, is termed static compliance (C_{Lstat}). Compliance is often measured during quiet breathing, also with an esophageal balloon-catheter system. During a breath, there are two times when airflow is zero. These occur at the end of inspiration and the end of expiration. The difference in Ppl at these two times also defines a change in elastic recoil pressure. This ΔPpl divided into the volume change is called the dynamic compliance of the lung (C_{Ldyn}).

In normal adult subjects, C_{Lstat} and C_{Ldyn} are nearly the same and range from 0.150 to 0.250 L/cm H_2O. In this group C_L varies directly with lung size, compliance being lower in subjects with small lungs.

Compliance is reduced in subjects with pulmonary fibrosis, often to values as low as 0.050 L/cm H_2O, reflecting the fact that these lungs are very stiff. Large changes in pressure produce only small changes in volume. Again, static and dynamic compliance are similar.

The situation in chronic obstructive pulmonary disease (COPD), especially emphysema, is different. Static compliance is much increased, to values often more than 0.500 L/cm H_2O. This high compliance reflects the floppy, inelastic lungs. However, C_{Ldyn} is much lower, often in the normal range. The explanation for this apparent paradox relates to the very nonuniform ventilation of the lungs in COPD, as discussed in Chapter 8. In essence, during breathing in COPD, air preferentially flows into and out of the more normal regions of the lung. Because the elasticity of these regions is not as severely impaired, C_{Ldyn} is nearer normal values. This difference between C_{Lstat} and C_{Ldyn} is referred to as frequency dependence of compliance. It is important to remember that a low C_{Ldyn} in COPD does not mean that the lung is stiff or fibrotic.

7C. RESPIRATORY SYSTEM COMPLIANCE

The compliance of the entire respiratory system (Crs) can also be measured. It requires that the respiratory muscles be relaxed. This measurement is most often made when a patient is on a ventilator. The patient's lungs are inflated, the airway is occluded, and the occluded airway pressure is measured. The lungs are allowed to deflate a measured amount, and a second occlusion pressure is obtained. Crs is the change in volume divided by the difference in the two pressures. Because the lungs and chest wall are in series, Crs includes both lung (C_{Lstat}) and chest wall compliance (Ccw). Because the reciprocals of the compliances are added, the equation describing this relationship is as follows:

$$\frac{1}{Crs} = \frac{1}{C_{LStat}} + \frac{1}{Ccw} \qquad \text{(Eq. 1)}$$

Thus, a decrease in Crs may be due to a decrease in either lung or chest wall compliance (or both), a fact that is sometimes overlooked.

7D. PATHOPHYSIOLOGY OF LUNG MECHANICS

The basics of lung mechanics have been presented. This section details the mechanical handicaps associated with obstructive and restrictive lung diseases.

Lung Static Elastic Recoil Pressure

We noted previously that the Ppl measured when the lung is not moving is the static elastic recoil pressure of the lung, which we now define as Pst. This pressure is measured from a small balloon placed in the lower esophagus.

In Figure 7-7, Pst is plotted during deflation of the lung from total lung capacity to residual volume. Three cases are shown: a normal subject (N); a patient with emphysema, an obstructive disorder (E); and a patient with pulmonary fibrosis, a restrictive disease (F). The curves are plotted as a function of absolute lung volume. Note the loss of lung recoil and hyperinflation in emphysema (E). This contrasts with the reduced lung volume and increased lung recoil in pulmonary fibrosis (F).

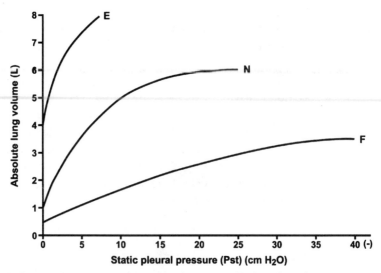

FIG. 7-7.   Lung static elastic recoil pressure (Pst) is plotted against absolute lung volume for three typical subjects: a patient with emphysema (E), a normal subject (N), and a patient with pulmonary fibrosis (F).

The E curve emphasizes two problems faced by the patient with emphysema and by most patients with COPD. First, the loss of recoil pressure means that the lung parenchyma cannot distend the airways as much as in the normal case (see the tethering springs in Fig. 2-2, page 8). Second, as shown in Figure 9-2, (page 94) the ability of the inspiratory muscles to generate force is reduced because of the hyperinflation.

In the F curve, representing the subject with pulmonary fibrosis, the ability of the expiratory muscles to develop force is reduced (see Fig. 9-2) because of the reduced lung volume. In addition, the increased recoil of the fibrotic lung requires the respiratory muscles to exert greater than normal force to expand the lung.

> **PEARL:** You might think that the Pst derives from the elastic and collagen fibers in the lung. However, the major contribution to the elastic recoil comes from surface tension forces acting at the air-fluid interface in the alveoli. This is demonstrated in Figure 7-8, in which are plotted static inflation and deflation airway pressures in a lung containing air (the normal situation) and the same lung inflated and deflated with

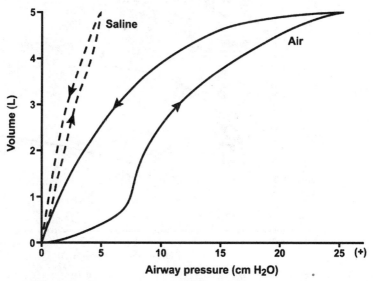

FIG. 7-8. Plot of static airway pressure versus lung volume in an excised lung first inflated and deflated with air. The arrows indicate the inflation and deflation paths. The lung is then degassed (all the air is removed) and inflated and deflated with saline. The marked shift to the left of the saline curve reflects the loss of recoil when surface tension at the alveolar air-fluid interface is abolished. The difference between the inflation-deflation curves is called hysteresis.

saline after the air has been removed. With saline filling, the alveolar air-fluid interface is abolished, as is the surface tension. Note how little recoil pressure remains in the saline lung, and what does remain reflects the relatively small tissue contribution. The markedly different inflation and deflation curves, especially in the air-filled lung, represent hysteresis—a common property of biologic tissues.

Work of Breathing

Figure 7-9 illustrates the effects of the alterations in Pst and in airflow resistance on the work of breathing required of the respiratory muscles. The static curves of Figure 7-7 have been replotted; the Ppl during inspiration has been added to each curve. Work is a product of pressure and volume. In each case, the hatched area between the inspiratory loop (identified by the *arrows*) and the static curve represents the resistive work of that breath. It is much increased in the E curve. The area between the static curve and the zero pressure axis reflects the work required to keep the lung inflated, i.e., the elastic work. Compared with the normal

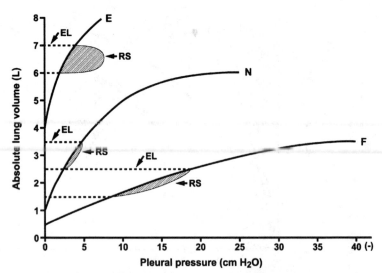

FIG. 7-9.   The pleural pressure generated during an inspiratory breath is plotted for a normal subject (N), a patient with emphysema (E), and a patient with fibrosis (F). The inspiratory loops are plotted on the static recoil curves of Figure 7-7. The hatched areas reflect the work of breathing required to overcome the resistance to airflow (RS). The areas between the static curve and the zero-pressure line reflect the work required to keep the lung inflated, the elastic work (EL). See text for further discussion.

curve, the subject with emphysema has large increases in work due to increased airflow resistance, whereas the subject with fibrosis has large increases in elastic work due to the stiffness of the lung. Although the total inspiratory work loop is less in emphysema than in fibrosis, more work is required during expiration. In addition, the hyperinflation in emphysema puts the system at a distinct mechanical disadvantage.

Static Lung Recoil Pressure and Maximal Expiratory Flow

In section 2B (page 6) and Figure 2-2 (page 8), we noted that lung elasticity, specifically Pst, is the pressure that drives maximal expiratory flow. It is informative to evaluate the relationship between maximal expiratory flow and Pst. Figure 7-10A shows how this relationship is obtained, and Figure 7-10B shows its behavior in normal and diseased lungs.

In Figure 7-10A, flow-volume and static lung recoil curves for a normal subject and a patient with pure emphysema are plotted on the common vertical axis of absolute lung volume. Thus, at

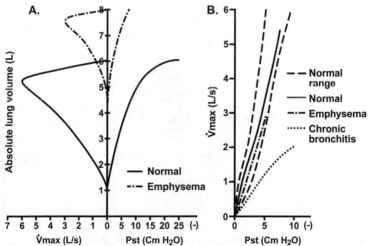

FIG. 7-10. Relationships between maximal expiratory flow (V̇max) and lung static elastic recoil pressure (Pst). **A.** V̇max and Pst are plotted on a common vertical absolute volume axis for a normal subject and a patient with pure emphysema. **B.** Corresponding values of V̇max and Pst obtained at various lung volumes are plotted with V̇max as a function of Pst. This is called a maximal flow static recoil curve. In the case of chronic bronchitis, the flow-volume and Pst-volume curves are not shown. See text for further discussion.

any lung volume corresponding to the decreasing portion of the flow-volume curve, it is possible to measure simultaneous values of maximal expiratory flow ($\dot{V}$max) and Pst.

In Figure 7-10B, Pst is plotted against $\dot{V}$max at various lung volumes. Such a graph is called a maximal flow static recoil (MFSR) curve. The normal range of values is shown by the two dashed lines. Values obtained from the normal curve in Figure 7-10A are connected by the solid line. The same has been done for the case of pure emphysema. Because the subject has no airway disease, the values fall within the normal range. This indicates that the decrease in maximal flow is mainly due to loss of lung recoil. However, if there is significant chronic bronchitis, the MFSR curve is shifted down and to the right, indicating that although there may be some loss of recoil pressure, this does not explain the decrease in flow, which is largely due to airway disease and associated increased airway resisitance. The MFSR cuve is useful in that it stresses the fact that maximal expiratory flow may be reduced by a loss of recoil pressure or significant airway disease or by both.

8

Distribution of Ventilation

Various pathologic processes alter the normal pattern of ventilation distribution (that is, the way an inhaled breath is distributed throughout the lung). For this reason, tests that detect abnormal patterns of ventilation distribution are fairly nonspecific and rarely of diagnostic importance. Their major contribution is that such abnormal patterns almost always are associated with alterations in ventilation-perfusion relationships (see page 66). Abnormal distribution of ventilation also contributes to the frequency dependence of compliance (see page 81).

There are several tests of ventilation distribution. Some are complex and require sophisticated equipment and complex analysis. This chapter discusses only the simplest procedure, the single-breath nitrogen (SBN$_2$) test.

8A. SINGLE-BREATH NITROGEN TEST

Procedure

The testing equipment and procedure are illustrated in Figure 8-1. The subject exhales to residual volume (RV) and then inhales a full breath of 100% oxygen from the bag on the left. A slow, complete exhalation is directed by the one-way valve through the orifice past the nitrogen meter into the spirometer. The orifice ensures that expiratory flow will be steady and slow (<0.5 L/s), and we recommend its use. The nitrogen meter continuously records the nitrogen concentration of the expired gas as it enters the spirometer. With simultaneous plotting of the expired nitrogen concentration

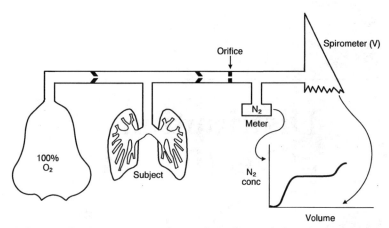

FIG. 8-1. Equipment required to perform the single-breath nitrogen washout test. A plot of exhaled nitrogen concentration (N_2 conc) against exhaled volume is shown at the lower right.

against expired volume on an X-Y plotter, the normal graph shown in Figure 8-1 and in Figure 8-2A is obtained.

Normal Results

The plot in Figure 8-2A is from a seated normal subject. There are four important portions of the normal graph: phases I through IV.

To understand this graph, we need to consider how the inhaled oxygen is normally distributed in the lungs of a seated subject. At RV, the alveolar nitrogen concentration can be considered uniform throughout the lung and alveolar gas is present in the trachea and upper airway (Fig. 8-3A). At RV, the alveoli (circles in Fig. 8-3A) in the more gravitationally dependent regions of the lung are at a smaller volume than those in the apical portions. Thus, the superior alveoli contain a larger volume of nitrogen at the same concentration. Therefore, as the subject inhales 100% oxygen, the superior alveoli receive proportionately less oxygen than the more dependent alveoli and the alveolar nitrogen is less diluted than in the dependent regions. Therefore, the nitrogen concentration is higher in the apical region. The result is a gradual decrease in nitrogen concentration further down the lung, and the most diluted alveolar gas is at the base (Fig. 8-3B). At the end of inspiration, the trachea and upper airway contain only oxygen.

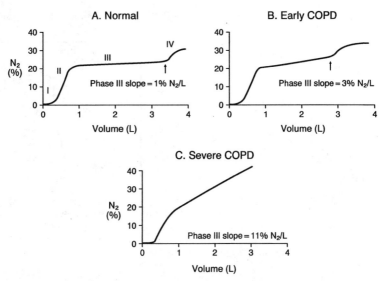

FIG. 8-2. Results of single-breath nitrogen washout tests on a normal subject (**A**), a subject with early chronic obstructive pulmonary disease (COPD; **B**), and a subject with an advanced case of COPD (**C**). Closing volume (when present) is identified by an arrow. The various phases are identified on **A**. The slope of phase III is given below each curve.

The events during expiration in the normal subject (Fig. 8-2*A*) are as follows. The initial gas passing the nitrogen meter comes from the trachea and upper airway and contains 100% oxygen. Thus, phase I shows 0% nitrogen. As expiration continues during phase II, alveolar gas begins washing out the dead space oxygen and the nitrogen concentration gradually increases.

Phase III consists entirely of alveolar gas. During a slow expiration, initially gas comes predominantly from the dependent alveolar regions, where the nitrogen concentration is lowest. As expiration continues, increasing amounts of gas come from the more superior regions, where nitrogen concentrations are higher. This sequence of events produces a gradually increasing nitrogen concentration during phase III. The normal slope of phase III is 1.0 to 2.5% nitrogen per liter expired. This value increases in the elderly.

An abrupt increase in nitrogen concentration occurs at the onset of phase IV. This reflects the gradual cessation of emptying of the dependent regions of the lung. Thus, more and more of the final expiration comes from the apical regions with the higher percentage

A. Residual Volume   B. Maximal Inspiration

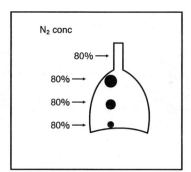
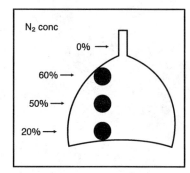

FIG. 8-3.   Normal distribution of a breath of oxygen inhaled from residual volume and the resulting gravity-dependent alveolar nitrogen concentration. **A.** Lung at residual volume. **B.** Lung after a maximal inspiration to total lung capacity.

of nitrogen. The onset of phase IV has been said to indicate the onset of airway closure in the dependent regions and is often called the "closing volume." However, whether airway closure actually occurs at this volume is still debatable. Normally, phase IV occurs with approximately 15% of the vital capacity still remaining. This value increases during normal aging, up to values of 25% vital capacity.

8B. CHANGES IN THE SINGLE-BREATH NITROGEN TEST IN DISEASE

With the onset of obstructive lung disease, the SBN_2 test is altered in two ways (Fig. 8-2B). The volume at which phase IV occurs (closing volume) increases. In addition, the slope of phase III increases. This occurs because the normal pattern of gas distribution, including the vertical gradient of nitrogen concentration described previously, is gradually abolished. Disease occurs unevenly throughout the lung. Regions of greater disease with high airway flow resistance empty less completely and hence receive less oxygen, and thus their nitrogen concentration is well above normal levels. Because the diseased areas empty more slowly than the more normal regions, the slope of phase III is greatly increased.

In advanced obstructive disease (Fig. 8-2C), there is no longer a phase IV. It becomes lost in the very steep slope of phase III.

8C. INTERPRETATION OF THE SINGLE-BREATH NITROGEN TEST

The more nonuniform the distribution of ventilation, the steeper the slope of phase III. There are associated increases in the nonuniformity of the perfusion of the alveolar capillaries. The impact of these changes on arterial blood gases is noted in section 6A, page 63.

It was thought that the increase in phase IV volume would be a useful, sensitive indicator of early airway disease. Unfortunately, it was not, and phase IV is rarely measured now. However, for many years phase III has been recognized as an excellent index of nonuniform ventilation. As shown in Figure 8-2, with the progress of obstructive airway disease, the slope of phase III progressively increases.

However, any measure of ventilation distribution is nonspecific. Increases in phase III are not limited to cases of airway obstruction. Increases also occur in pulmonary fibrosis, congestive heart failure, sarcoidosis, and other conditions in which airway disease is not the principal abnormality.

In conclusion, consideration of the distribution of ventilation tells much about lung physiology. Disorders of ventilation distribution are extremely important in the pathophysiology of conditions such as chronic bronchitis, asthma, and emphysema. In terms of the clinical evaluation of the patient with lung disease or unexplained dyspnea, however, tests of ventilation distribution add very little to a basic battery of spirometry and tests of lung volumes, diffusing capacity, and arterial blood gases.

9

Maximal Respiratory Pressures

In some clinical situations, evaluation of the strength of the respiratory muscles is very helpful. The strength of skeletal muscles, such as those of the arm, is easily tested by determining the force that they can develop, as by lifting weights. In contrast, the strength of the respiratory muscles can be determined by measuring the pressures developed against an occluded airway.

9A. PHYSIOLOGIC PRINCIPLES

Some basic muscle physiology is reviewed here to aid in determining the best way of estimating the strength of respiratory muscles. Muscles, when maximally stimulated at different lengths, exhibit a characteristic length-tension behavior, as depicted in Figure 9-1. The greatest tension developed by the muscle occurs when it is at its optimal physiologic length. Less tension is developed at other lengths. To apply this concept to respiratory muscles, volume can be thought of as equivalent to length and pressure as equivalent to tension. The *expiratory* muscles (chest wall and abdominal muscles) are at their optimal lengths near total lung capacity. Figure 9-2 shows, as expected, that the highest expiratory pressures are generated near total lung capacity. The subject blows as hard as possible against an occluded airway. Conversely, near residual volume, the *inspiratory* muscles (primarily the diaphragm) are at their optimal lengths. Near residual volume, they develop the most negative pressure when the subject is sucking against an occluded airway. Therefore, the maximal strength of the expiratory muscles is

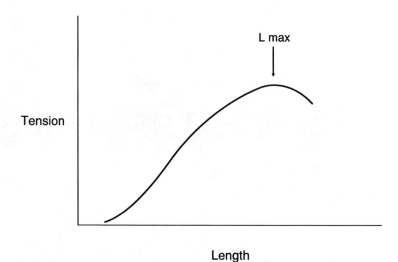

FIG. 9-1.   Classic length-tension behavior of striated muscle. L max is the length at which maximal tension can be developed.

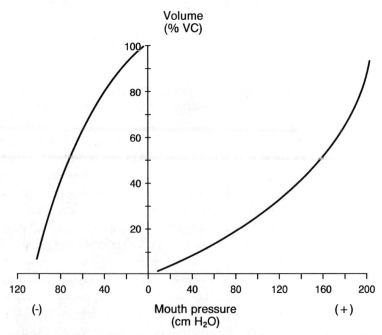

FIG. 9-2.   Maximal respiratory pressure that can be developed statically at various lung volumes (vital capacity, VC). Expiratory pressures are positive, and inspiratory pressures are negative. Total lung capacity is at 100% VC and residual volume at 0% VC.

measured near total lung capacity and that of the inspiratory muscles is measured near residual volume.

9B. MEASUREMENT TECHNIQUES

The device we use is shown in Figure 9-3. It consists of a hollow stainless-steel tube to which are attached negative- and positive-pressure gauges. The distal end of the tube is occluded, except for a 2-mm hole.

Maximal expiratory pressure (PEmax) is measured as follows. The subject inhales maximally, holds the rubber tubing firmly against the mouth, and exhales as hard as possible. Several reproducible efforts are obtained, and the highest positive pressure maintained for 0.9 second is recorded. Rubber tubing held firmly against the lips is used rather than a mouthpiece because at high pressures (150 cm H_2O or more) air leaks around a conventional mouthpiece, the buccal muscles not being strong enough to maintain a tight seal. A nose clip is not used.

Maximal inspiratory pressure (PImax) is measured by having the subject exhale to residual volume, hold the rubber tubing against the lips, and suck as hard as possible. Again, the highest negative pressure sustained for 2 seconds is recorded. The small 2-mm hole at the distal end ensures that the device is measuring the alveolar pressure developed in the lung by the inspiratory muscles. If the subject closes the glottis and sucks with the cheeks, a high negative pressure can be developed. The leak prevents this from happening because the pressure produced by sucking with a closed glottis decreases rapidly and cannot be sustained for 0.9 second. To be accurate, the subject must exert maximal effort. Herein lies a shortcoming of the test. These efforts can be uncomfortable. Some subjects are unable, or unwilling, to make such effort. Determined coaching by the technician is essential.

9C. NORMAL VALUES

Normal values obtained from a motivated group of 60 normal male and 60 normal female subjects are listed in Table 9-1. As anticipated from Figure 9-2, PEmax is roughly double the PImax. Male subjects developed greater pressures than female subjects, and both sexes

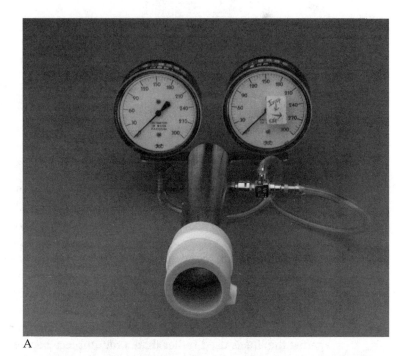

A

B

FIG. 9-3. Instrument used to measure maximal static expiratory and inspiratory pressures. The expiratory gauge measures 0 to +300 cm H_2O, and the inspiratory gauge 0 to −300 cm H_2O. Gauges are alternately connected to the cylinder by a three-way stopcock, as indicated by the arrows on the right-hand gauge (**A**). The side view (**B**) shows the small 2-mm hole at the distal end of the metal tube.

TABLE 9-1. Normal values for maximal respiratory pressures, by age

Pressure	Age (yr)				
	20–54	55–59	60–64	65–69	70–74
PImax, cm H_2O*					
Male	-124 ± 44	-103 ± 32	-103 ± 32	-103 ± 32	-103 ± 32
Female	-87 ± 32	-77 ± 26	-73 ± 26	-70 ± 26	-65 ± 26
PEmax, cm H_2O*					
Male	233 ± 84	218 ± 74	209 ± 74	197 ± 74	185 ± 74
Female	152 ± 54	145 ± 40	140 ± 40	135 ± 40	128 ± 40

PEmax, maximal expiratory pressure; PImax, maximal inspiratory pressure.
*Numbers represent mean $\pm$ 2 standard deviations.

had a decline in pressure with age, except for inspiratory pressures in male subjects.

9D. INDICATIONS FOR MAXIMAL PRESSURE MEASUREMENTS

1. In patients with neuromuscular disease who have dyspnea, measurement of respiratory muscle strength is useful. We studied 10 subjects with early neuromuscular diseases (amyotrophic lateral sclerosis, myasthenia gravis, and polymyositis). Eight of the 10 had significant dyspnea, but only two had a significant reduction in the vital capacity (77%). Five had a reduced maximal voluntary ventilation (73%). However, nine patients had significant reductions in PEmax (47% predicted) and PImax (34% predicted). In the early stages, dyspnea was best explained by a reduction in respiratory muscle strength at a time when the strength of other skeletal muscles was little impaired. Table 9-2 lists some neuromuscular

TABLE 9-2. Neuromuscular disorders associated with respiratory muscle weakness

Amyotrophic lateral sclerosis	Guillain-Barré syndrome
Myasthenia gravis	Syringomyelia
Muscular dystrophy	Parkinson's disease
Polymyositis	Steroid myopathy
Poliomyelitis, postpolio syndrome	Polyneuropathy
Stroke	Spinal cord injury
Diaphragm paralysis	Acid maltase deficiency

conditions in which respiratory muscle weakness has been encountered.

2. It is useful to measure respiratory muscle strength in the co-operative subject with an isolated, unexplained decrease in the vital capacity or maximal voluntary ventilation. Such decreases could be early signs of respiratory muscle weakness and could explain a complaint of dyspnea. Other conditions in which muscle weakness has been documented are lupus erythematosus, lead poisoning, scleroderma, and hyperthyroidism.

PEARLS: An effective cough is generally not possible when maximal expiratory pressure is less than 40 cm H_2O.

Unexplained fainting may be due to cough syncope in the subject with severe chronic bronchitis. Sustained airway pressures of more than 300 cm H_2O have been measured in this condition during paroxysms of coughing. Such pressures are sufficient to reduce venous return and thus cardiac output, leading to syncope, occasionally even when the subject is supine.

3. Measurement of respiratory muscle strength in the intensive care unit has been advocated as an assessment of readiness to wean from mechanical ventilation. A pressure transducer can be connected to the 15-mm adapter on the endotracheal tube. If testing is performed for patients who are not intu-bated (as a measure of risk of respiratory failure in patients with respiratory muscle weakness), it is important to have the small leak in the device described in section 9B.

When maximal respiratory pressures are used for assessment of weaning potential, an inspiratory pressure lower than −20 cm H_2O and an expiratory pressure more than +50 cm H_2O have been identified as predictive of the ability to wean most patients from ventilatory support. However, use of a single factor in deciding about weaning potential is not encouraged. It must be kept in mind that the ability to breathe unassisted depends on the balance between the capacity of the respiratory muscles to perform work and the workload imposed on the respiratory muscles by the chest wall and lungs.

10

Preoperative Pulmonary Function Testing

The goals of preoperative pulmonary function testing are (1) to detect unrecognized lung disease, (2) to estimate the risk of operation compared with the potential benefit, (3) to plan perioperative care, and (4) to estimate postoperative lung function. Several studies have shown a high prevalence of unsuspected impairment of lung function in surgical patients and suggest that preoperative pulmonary function testing is underutilized. There is evidence that appropriate perioperative management improves surgical outcome in patients with impaired lung function.

10A. WHO SHOULD BE TESTED?

The indications for testing depend on the characteristics of the patient and on the planned surgical procedure. Table 10-1 lists the characteristics of the patient and the surgical procedures for which testing is recommended. We believe that preoperative testing should be done on all patients scheduled for any lung resection. We also recommend testing before upper abdominal and thoracic operation in patients with known lung disease and for smokers older than 40 (up to one-fourth of such smokers have abnormal lung function) because these procedures present the greatest risk for patients with impaired lung function. When a significant abnormality is detected, appropriate perioperative intervention may reduce the morbidity and mortality related to operation. Such

TABLE 10-1.   Indications for preoperative pulmonary function testing

Subject
    Known pulmonary dysfunction
    Current smoking, especially if >1 pack per day
    Chronic productive cough
    Recent respiratory infection
    Advanced age
    Obesity >30% over ideal weight
    Thoracic cage deformity, such as kyphoscoliosis
    Neuromuscular disease, such as amyotrophic lateral sclerosis or
        myasthenia gravis
Procedure
    Thoracic or upper abdominal operation
    Pulmonary resection
    Prolonged anesthesia

intervention includes use of bronchodilators and postoperative use of incentive spirometry. Although the benefit of smoking cessation before operation has not been proved, it is common practice to recommend that smokers, especially those with impaired lung function, stop smoking preoperatively.

10B. WHAT TESTS SHOULD BE DONE?

For patients with obstructive disorders, spirometry before and after bronchodilator therapy may be sufficient preoperative testing. However, for those with moderate to severe airway obstruction, arterial carbon dioxide tension should also be measured. Table 10-2 lists general guidelines for interpreting the test results in terms of risk to the patient.

TABLE 10-2.   Guidelines for estimating postoperative risks

Test	Increased risk	High risk
FVC	<50% predicted	≤1.5 L
FEV_1	<2.0 L or <50% predicted	<1.0 L
MVV		<50% predicted
$Paco_2$		≥45 mm Hg

FEV_1, forced expiratory volume in 1 second; FVC, forced vital capacity; MVV, maximal voluntary ventilation; $Paco_2$, arterial tension of carbon dioxide.

The risk of surgical procedures for patients with restrictive disorders has not been as well studied as that for patients with obstructive disorders. We recommend following similar guidelines, but keeping in mind the cause of restriction (lung parenchymal disease, chest wall disorders, muscle weakness, obesity).

Indications for measurement of the diffusing capacity of the lungs (D_{LCO}) are not clearly established. We recommend that the D_{LCO} be measured in patients with restrictive disorders to evaluate the severity of gas exchange abnormality. This abnormality may be more severe than expected from the degree of ventilatory impairment alone.

Oximetry is an inexpensive measure of gas exchange but is relatively nonspecific and insensitive, even when performed during exercise. We do not recommend its use for determining operative risk. It is useful, however, for monitoring oxygen therapy postoperatively.

Maximal voluntary ventilation is also used as a predictor of postoperative respiratory complications. It is less reproducible than the forced expiratory volume in 1 second (FEV_1) and is more dependent on muscle strength and effort. For these reasons it is no longer used to determine a subject's eligibility for Social Security disability payments. However, it does have a role in preoperative assessment and seems to be comparable to the FEV_1 for predicting postoperative respiratory complications.

10C. ADDITIONAL STUDIES

Quantitative radionuclide scintigraphy has been used to determine regional ventilation and perfusion of the lungs. The results have been used to improve estimates of postoperative pulmonary function, especially for patients with marginal lung function.

Maximal cardiopulmonary exercise studies have been used for preoperative assessment. Several authors have reported low rates of postoperative complications in patients with a maximal oxygen uptake of more than 20 mL/kg/min and high rates of complications with a maximal oxygen uptake of less than 15 mL/kg/min. This form of testing requires sophisticated equipment and considerable technical expertise. It is therefore more expensive than other tests. Yet the cost of testing is small compared with that of most surgical procedures.

10D. WHAT IS PROHIBITIVE RISK?

Several algorithms have been developed for calculation of lung function after resection of lung tissue. One approach requires an estimation of the number of lung segments, out of a total of 18, that are likely to be removed. Then the following calculation is performed:

$$\text{Preoperative FEV}_1 \times \frac{(\text{no. of remaining segments})}{18} = \text{postoperative FEV}_1$$

(Eq. 1)

Thus, if five segments are to be removed and the preoperative FEV_1 is 2.0 L, the predicted postoperative FEV_1 is 1.4 L

$$(2 \times \frac{18 - 5}{18} = 1.4).$$

The postoperative FEV_1 predicted from this calculation is the estimated level of lung function after full recovery, not immediately after operation. A common recommendation is that surgical resection should not be performed if the predicted postoperative FEV_1 is less than 0.8 L. However, several recent studies suggest that this is not an absolute contraindication. Specialized centers with excellent perioperative care have reported low morbidity and mortality in severely impaired patients [1].

REFERENCE

1. Cerfolio RJ, Allen MS, Trastek VF, Deschamps C, Scanlon PD, Pairolero PC. Lung resection in patients with compromised pulmonary function. *Ann Thorac Surg* 62: 348–351, 1996.

11

Simple Tests of Exercise Capacity

In most instances the clinician has an estimate of a patient's exercise capacity. This is based on the history, results of physical examination, and pertinent data such as chest radiographs, electrocardiogram, blood cell count, and standard pulmonary function tests, possibly including arterial blood gas values.

However, in some situations a quantitative estimate of a patient's exercise capacity is needed. Before formal exercise studies are requested, some relatively simple tests can be performed. These can be done in the office or in a hospital's pulmonary function laboratory. They may obviate more extensive testing by providing a sufficient assessment of a patient's limitation.

11A. EXERCISE OXIMETRY

Pulse oximetry, available in most hospitals, is an inexpensive and noninvasive method of estimating arterial oxygen saturation in the absence of significant concentrations of abnormal hemoglobins. After an appropriate site for exercising is selected and the pulse oximetry quality assurance criteria are satisfied, the oxygen saturation at rest is recorded. If the resting saturation is normal or near normal, the subject exercises until he or she is short of breath. In some disease entities, such as pulmonary fibrosis, pulmonary hypertension, and emphysema, values at rest are normal but surprising desaturation is noted with exercise. In this situation, a wise step is to repeat the exercise with the patient breathing oxygen to determine whether the saturation is easily corrected and the dyspnea ameliorated.

If a patient's resting saturation is low, this may be all the information needed. If supplemental oxygen is to be prescribed, however, the flow rate of oxygen that will provide an adequate resting saturation and the flow needed to maintain adequate saturation with mild exertion may need to be determined.

For such studies, it is important that the distance and time walked be recorded. For prescribing oxygen, the levels of exercise (distance walked) can be compared without and with supplemental oxygen. In some patients with chronic obstructive pulmonary disease (COPD) and those with chest wall and neuromuscular limitations in whom carbon dioxide retention may be of concern, resting arterial blood gas values while the patient is breathing the prescribed oxygen concentration should be obtained. Determining arterial blood gas values during exercise while breathing the prescribed oxygen concentration is generally not necessary.

> **PEARL:** In a few situations, the saturation is falsely low when the pulse oximeter is used on the finger. These situations include thick calluses, excessive ambient light, use of bright shades of nail polish, jaundice, and conditions with poor peripheral circulation such as scleroderma and Raynaud's disease. In cases with a poor pulse signal, the earlobe is an alternative site. If there is any doubt about the reliability of the oximeter readings, or if the reading does not match the clinical situation, arterial blood gas studies are recommended.

11B. WALKING TESTS: 6- AND 12-MINUTE

These simple walking tests are useful for quantifying and documenting over time a patient's exercise capacity. They can be utilized in both pulmonary and cardiac disease with reasonable precautions. They are also valuable for quantifying the progress of patients in rehabilitation programs [1].

The tests are best performed in a building with unobstructed, level corridors. A distance of 100 ft can be measured and the number of laps counted. Neither test is superior over the other. Because the 6-minute test is less demanding, it is used more often, especially in very sick patients. The subject is instructed to walk back and forth over the course and go as far as possible in 6 minutes. The subject should be encouraged by standardized statements such as "You're doing well" or "Keep up the good work." Subjects are allowed to stop and rest during the test but are asked to resume

TABLE 11-1.   Relation of 6- and 12-minute walks to speed

	Distance (ft) walked in:	
Speed (mph)	6 min	12 min
3	1,584	3,168
2	1,056	2,112
1	528	1,056
0.5	264	528
0.25	132	264

Prediction equations for the distance walked during the 6-minute (6MWD) test for adults of ages 40 to 80 years. Results are given in meters (1 meter = 3.28 ft) [2]. Men: 6MWD = (7.57 × height cm) − (5.02 × age yr) − (1.76 × weight kg) − 309 meters. Women: 6MWD = (2.11 × height cm) − (5.78 × age yr) − (2.29 × weight kg) + 667 meters (2).

walking as soon as possible. Pulse rate is recorded before and after the test. Ideally, the test is repeated after a 10- to 15-minute rest, and the greatest distance walked is recorded. If the patient is receiving oxygen, the flow rate and mode of transport, such as carried or pulled unit, is recorded.

Table 11-1 relates the distances walked to the average rate of walking in miles per hour. Recently, prediction equations for the 6-minute test have become available for average healthy adults of ages 40 to 80 years. These are listed in Table 11-1. The use of the test is twofold. First, by comparing your patient's results with the predicted norm, you gain an estimate of the patient's degree of impairment. Second, the test is most valuable as a measure of the patient's response to therapy or the progression of disease.

11C. STAIR-CLIMBING TEST

For many years, physicians have used stair climbing to estimate a patient's cardiopulmonary reserve. The empirical nature of stair climbing has been a drawback. However, in a recent study subjects with COPD climbed stairs until they became limited by symptoms and stopped [3]. A significant correlation was found between the number of steps climbed and (1) peak oxygen consumption and (2) maximal exercise ventilation. This test is another way to estimate operative risk in patients with COPD who are to undergo thoracic operation. The study found that, on average, the ability to climb 83 steps was equivalent to a maximal oxygen consumption ($\dot{V}o_2$max) of 20 mL/kg/min. The ability to reach a maximal oxygen consumption of 20 mL/kg/min has been reported to be associated with fewer complications after lung resection or thoracotomy.

Stair climbing is more cumbersome than the 6- or 12-minute walk. However, it does push most patients closer to their maximal oxygen consumption, $\dot{V}o_2$max, an end point of greater physiologic significance.

11D. VENTILATORY RESERVE

Measuring a subject's ventilation during a given task or exercise provides an estimate of the demand of that task. There are simple ways of measuring minute ventilation. We and others have found that reconditioned gas meters (such as used by gas companies) are accurate. By means of a two-way valve, expired air is directed through the meter. The revolution of the meter dial can be converted to liters per minute.

The definition of ventilatory reserve (VR) is given by this relationship:

$$VR = \frac{MVV - \text{exercise ventilation} (\dot{V}E)}{MVV} \times 100 \qquad \text{(Eq. 1)}$$

Given a maximal voluntary ventilation (MVV) of 60 L/min and an exercise ventilation ($\dot{V}E$) of 30 L/min during a given task, the VR is 50% $\left(\frac{60-30}{60}\right)$. The greater the $\dot{V}E$, the lower the reserve and the more likely it is that the patient will become dyspneic. A VR of less than 50% is usually associated with dyspnea. Another approach is to subtract $\dot{V}E$ from the MVV. A value of MVV $-$ $\dot{V}E$ less than 20 L/min indicates severe ventilatory limitation.

11E. RATING OF RESPIRATORY IMPAIRMENT

Another approach to estimating respiratory impairment is based on the percentage reduction in various pulmonary function tests. One recommendation presented by the American Thoracic Society is summarized in Table 11-2. It provides useful guidelines. If a

TABLE 11-2. Estimations of respiratory impairment based on results of pulmonary function tests

Condition	Test*				
	FVC	FEV_1	FEV_1/FVC	$D_{L_{CO}}$	$\dot{V}O_2max$
Normal	>80	>80	>75	>80	>75
Mild impairment	60–80	60–80	60–75	60–80	60–75
Moderate impairment (unable to meet physical requirements of many jobs)	50–60	40–60	40–60	40–60	40–60
Severe impairment (unable to meet most job demands, including travel to work)	<50	<40	<40	<40	<40

*All tests relate to the percentage of the normal predicted value for an individual.
$D_{L_{CO}}$, diffusing capacity of carbon monoxide; FEV_1, forced expiratory volume in 1 second; FVC, forced vital capacity; $\dot{V}O_2max$, maximal oxygen consumption.
Data from Ad Hoc Committee on Impairment/Disability Evaluation: Evaluation of impairment/disability secondary to respiratory disorders. *Am Rev Respir Dis* 133:1205–1209, 1986.

patient complains of severe dyspnea but the tests show only mild to moderate impairment, causes other than respiratory should be sought. If none exist, cardiopulmonary exercise testing might be appropriate.

11F. CARDIOPULMONARY EXERCISE TESTING

Cardiopulmonary exercise testing requires sophisticated equipment and should be performed only by laboratories with strict quality control, experienced physiologic direction, appropriate medical supervision, and considerable experience in doing such tests [4]. Numerous variables of gas exchange and cardiac function, often requiring an indwelling arterial catheter for repeated blood gas determinations, are measured. The measurements include ventilation, oxygen consumption ($\dot{V}O_2$), carbon dioxide production ($\dot{V}CO_2$), dead space ventilation, and alveolar-arterial oxygen gradients. In some laboratories, $\dot{V}O_2$ and $\dot{V}CO_2$ are measured breath by breath. Also measured are the heart rate, blood pressure, and lactate levels, and electrocardiography is performed.

Some of the indications for cardiopulmonary exercise testing are as follows:

1. To distinguish between cardiac and pulmonary causes of dyspnea in complex cases
2. To determine whether the patient's symptoms are due to deconditioning
3. To detect the malingering patient
4. To provide disability evaluation in problem cases
5. To determine whether the subject can meet the work requirements of a given occupation

REFERENCES

1. Crapo RO, Casaburi R, Coates AL, et al. ATS statement: Guidelines for the six-minute walk test. *Am J Respir Crit Care Med* 166:111–117, 2002.
2. Enright PL, Sherrill DL. Reference equations for the six-minute walk in healthy adults. *Am J Respir Crit Care Med* 158:1384–1387, 1998.
3. Pollock M, Roa J, Benditt J, Celli B. Estimation of ventilatory reserve by stair climbing: A study in patients with chronic airflow obstruction. *Chest* 104:1378–1383, 1993.
4. Jones NL, Killian KJ. Exercise limitation in health and disease. *N Engl J Med* 343:632–641, 2000.

12

Patterns in Various Diseases

There are patterns of pulmonary function test abnormalities that are typical for most subjects with a particular disease. Table 12-1 expands on Table 3-1, adding data on lung volumes, arterial blood gas values, diffusing capacity, lung compliance and resistance, the single-breath nitrogen test, and maximal respiratory pressures. It should be emphasized that a clinical diagnosis is not made from these test results alone. Rather they quantify the lung impairment and are to be interpreted in the context of the total clinical picture. For this discussion, obstructive disease is categorized into four conditions: Emphysema, chronic bronchitis, chronic obstructive pulmonary disease, and asthma. Restrictive conditions are divided into those due to pulmonary parenchymal disease and extrapulmonary causes.

12A. EMPHYSEMA

Pure emphysema (such as α_1-antitrypsin deficiency) is associated with hyperinflation (increased total lung capacity [TLC]); a significant loss of lung elasticity (decreased recoil pressure at TLC and increased static compliance of the lung [PTLC and C_{Lstat}]); and often a substantial decrease in the diffusing capacity of the lung (DL_{CO}, reflecting destruction of alveoli). Resting arterial tension of oxygen (Pao_2) and carbon dioxide ($Paco_2$) are generally normal unless the condition is far advanced. Bullae, predominantly in the lower lung fields, are typical in α_1-antitrypsin deficiency.

TABLE 12-1. Patterns of pulmonary function tests in disease

Test	Units	Emphysema	Chronic bronchitis	Chronic obstructive pulmonary disease	Asthma	Restrictive Intra-pulmonary	Restrictive Extra-pulmonary	Neuro-muscular disease	Congestive heart failure	Obesity
FVC	L	(N)→↓	(N)→↓	(N)→↓	→↓	→↓	→↓	N→↓	→↓	N→↓
FEV₁	L	↓	→	→	→	N→↓	→↓	N→↓	→↓	N→↓
FEV₁/FVC	%	↓	→	→	N→↓	N→↑	N	N	N→↑	N
FEF₂₅₋₇₅	L/s	↓	→	→	→	N→↑	→	N→↓	→	N
PEF	L/min	↓	→	→	→	N→↑	→	N→↑	→	N→↓
MVV	L/min	↓	→	→	→	N→↑	→	N→↑	→	N→↓
FEF₅₀	L/s	↓	→	→	→	N	→	N→↓	→	N
Slope of FV curve		↓	↓	↓						
TLC	L	→	→N→↑	→N→↓	N→↑	←→→N	N→↑	N→↑	N→↑	N→↑
RV	L	←↑	←↑	←↑	N→↑	→→N	→→↓	N→↑	↑→N→↑	↑→N→↑
RV/TLC	%	←↑	←↑	←↑	←	N	N→↑	N→↑	↑→N→↑	→→N→↑
DLco	mL/mm Hg/min	→	N→↑	N→↑	↑→N→↓	N→↑	N	N→↑	↑→N→↑	→→N→↓
DL/VA	mL/mm Hg/min/L	→	N→↑	N→↑	↑→N→↑	N→↑	N	N	→	N→↑

Pao₂	torr*	N→↓		N→↓	N→↓	N→↓↑	→	N	N→↓	N→↓
Sao₂	%	N→↓		N→↑	N→↑	N→↑	→	N	N→↑	N→↑
Paco₂	torr*	N→↑		N→↑	N→↑	N→↑	→	N	N→↑	N
pH	−log[H+]	N→↓	↓	N→↓	N→↓	N→↓	→	N	N→↓	N
Raw	cm H₂O/L/s	↑	↑	↑	↑	↑	N→↑	N	N→↑	N
CL_stat	L/cm H₂O	↑	↑	↑	N→↑	N→↑	→	N	N→↑	N
CL_dyn	L/cm H₂O	→	→	N→↑	N→↑	→→	N→↑	N	N→↑	N
PTLC	cm H₂O	←	N→↑	N→↑	→	→	N→↑	N	N→↑	N
Phase III	% N₂/L	A	↔→A	↔→A	→	←	←	N	N→↑	N→↑
Phase IV	% vital capacity	A	↔→A	↔→A	→	←	←	N	N→↑	N→↑
PEmax	cm H₂O	N→↓	←	↓→N→↑	N	N	N→↑	N→↑	N	N
PImax	cm H₂O	→	N	N→↑	N	N	N→↑	N→↑	N	N

*torr, equivalent to mm Hg.

A, often absent; N, normal; (N), occasionally normal; →, to; ↑, increased; ↓, decreased; CL_dyn, dynamic compliance of the lung; CL_stat, static compliance of the lung; DL_CO, diffusing capacity of carbon monoxide; DL/VA, diffusing capacity of the lung/alveolar volume; FEF_{25-75}, forced expiratory flow rate over the middle 50% of the FVC; FEF_{50}, forced expiratory flow after 50% of the FVC has been exhaled; FEV₁, forced expiratory volume in 1 second; FV, flow-volume; FVC, forced vital capacity; MVV, maximal voluntary ventilation; Paco₂, arterial carbon dioxide tension; Pao₂, arterial oxygen tension; PEF, peak expiratory flow; PEmax, maximal expiratory pressure; PImax, maximal inspiratory pressure; PTLC, lung recoil pressure at TLC; Raw, airway resistance; RV, residual volume; Sao₂, arterial oxygen saturation; TLC, total lung capacity.

12B. CHRONIC BRONCHITIS

Pure chronic bronchitis is typically found in heavy cigarette smokers with a chronic productive cough and frequent respiratory infections. In contrast to emphysema, lung recoil is often normal but the Pao_2 may be low and associated with carbon dioxide retention (increased $Paco_2$).

12C. CHRONIC OBSTRUCTIVE PULMONARY DISEASE

The lungs of most smokers in whom obstructive lung disease develops show a mixture of emphysema and chronic bronchitis. The tests reflect contributions of both disease processes. For example, hyperinflation tends to be greater than in pure chronic bronchitis, but carbon dioxide retention may not be present.

12D. ASTHMA

Because lung function may be normal between attacks, the data in Table 12-1 reflect those during a moderate attack in a nonsmoker. The changes are much like those in chronic obstructive pulmonary disease, except for the tendency toward hyperventilation and respiratory alkalosis (increased pH, decreased $Paco_2$). Also, the response to bronchodilators (not shown in Table 12-1) is typically very striking. In remission, all test results, with the occasional exception of the residual volume/total lung capacity ratio (RV/TLC), may return to normal; however, the methacholine challenge test may still be positive. The ratio of forced expiratory volume in 1 second to forced vital capacity (FEV_1/FVC) may be normal, especially during a mild attack. The DL_{CO} may be normal, increased, or decreased.

12E. PULMONARY RESTRICTION

Idiopathic pulmonary fibrosis is the classic example of an intrapulmonary restrictive process. Peak expiratory flows may be normal or low, the diffusion capacity decreased, PTLC generally increased,

TABLE 12-2.   Causes of restrictive disease

Pulmonary
  Pulmonary fibrosis and interstitial pneumonitis
  Asbestosis
  Neoplasms, including lymphangitic carcinoma
  Pneumonia
  Sarcoidosis
  Bronchiolitis obliterans with organizing pneumonia (BOOP)
  Hypersensitivity pneumonitis
  Alveolar proteinosis
  Histiocytosis X (Langerhans' cell histiocytosis or eosinophilic
    granuloma)
  Lung resectional operation
  Atelectasis
Extrapulmonary
  Pleural cavity
    Pleural effusion
    Pneumothorax
    Fibrothorax
    Cardiac enlargement
  Neuromuscular
    Diaphragmatic paralysis
    Neuromuscular diseases, including amyotrophic lateral sclerosis,
      myasthenia gravis, polymyositis
  Chest wall
    Kyphoscoliosis
    Ankylosing spondylitis
    Thoracoplasty
    Ascites
    Pregnancy

lung compliance decreased, and the slope of the expiratory flow-volume curve steep.

Some other parenchymal conditions that cause restriction are listed in Table 12-2. However, not all of them always produce the classic picture described here. The slope of the flow-volume curve may not be increased and the lung recoil may not be altered, in part because restriction may be combined with obstruction. Examples are endobronchial involvement in sarcoid and tuberculosis. This mixed pattern is also frequent in cystic fibrosis and eosinophilic granuloma (histiocytosis X) and is striking in lymphangioleiomyomatosis.

12F. EXTRAPULMONARY RESTRICTION

In the case of extrapulmonary restriction, the lung parenchyma is assumed to be normal. The most frequent causes of this type of restriction are listed in Table 12-2. The main abnormalities are the decreased lung volumes with generally normal gas exchange. Because the DL_{CO} is somewhat volume-dependent, it may be reduced. Resection in an otherwise normal lung also fits this pattern.

Severe degrees of restriction, as in advanced kyphoscoliosis, can lead to respiratory insufficiency with abnormal gas exchange.

12G. NEUROMUSCULAR DISEASE

The hallmark of early neuromuscular disease is a decrease in respiratory muscle strength reflected in decreases in maximal expiratory and inspiratory pressures. At this stage, all other test results can be normal despite the patient complaining of exertional dyspnea. As the process progresses, the maximal voluntary ventilation is next to decrease, followed by decreases in the FVC and TLC with accompanying impairment of gas exchange. Ultimately, the picture fits that of a restrictive extrapulmonary disorder.

These patterns are most frequent in amyotrophic lateral sclerosis, myasthenia gravis, and polymyositis. They have also been noted in syringomyelia, muscular dystrophy, parkinsonism, various myopathies, and Guillain-Barré syndrome.

12H. CONGESTIVE HEART FAILURE

The effects of left-sided congestive heart failure with pulmonary congestion on the function of an otherwise normal lung are often not appreciated. In some cases, the predominant change is one of pure restriction with a normal FEV_1/FVC ratio, flows decreased in proportion to the FVC, and a normal flow-volume curve slope. The chest radiograph may suggest interstitial fibrosis.

In other cases, there may be a mixed restrictive-obstructive pattern with decreases in flow out of proportion to volume reduction. The FEV_1/FVC ratio is reduced, as is the slope of the flow-volume curve. The obstructive component is in part due to peribronchial edema, which narrows the airways and produces "cardiac asthma." Of interest, the result of the methacholine challenge test may be positive for reasons that are unclear.

In years past, the effectiveness of therapy for pulmonary congestion was sometimes monitored by measuring changes in the vital capacity. Congestive heart failure is highlighted here because it is often overlooked as a possible cause of a restrictive or obstructive pattern.

12I. OBESITY

A frequent question is whether the changes in the results of pulmonary function tests are explained by obesity. Data are sparse on obesity and pulmonary function in normal, nonsmoking subjects. One study [1] included otherwise normal, *nonsmoking*, massively obese subjects aged 19 to 32 years (mean, 25 yr). Subjects were categorized by their weight/height (kg/cm) ratio (normal, 0.5 or less). The ratios in the heaviest subjects ranged between 1.0 and 1.10. There was a progressive small *increase* in D_{CO} with increasing ratio. Only the heaviest subjects had decreases in TLC, vital capacity, and maximal voluntary ventilation to 79, 69, and 61% of predicted, respectively. Expiratory flows and FEV_1 remained normal. The study indicates that function is altered only with massive obesity (374 lb [170 kg] in a 5-ft 6-in. [168 cm] subject, for example) and only mildly in otherwise healthy young adults. However, the adverse effects of obesity may be greater in the elderly and in smokers. Indeed, in contrast to the study described above are the findings on the effect of weight gain on pulmonary function in older subjects with mild to moderate obstructive lung disease [2]. These subjects gained weight when they quit smoking. Men had a loss of FVC of 17.4 mL/kg gained and a loss of FEV_1 of 11.1 mL/kg of weight gained. Women showed similar but smaller changes, losing FVC at a rate of 10.6 mL/kg and FEV_1 at a rate of 5.6 mL/kg of weight gained.

REFERENCES

1. Ray CS, Sue DY, Bray G, Hansen JE, Wasserman K. Effects of obesity on respiratory function. *Am Rev Respir Dis* 128:501–506. 1983.
2. Wise RA, Enright PL, Connett JE, et al. Effect of weight gain on pulmonary function after smoking cessation in the Lung Health Study. *Am J Respir Crit Care Med* 157:866–872. 1998.

13

When to Test and What to Order

The recommendations for *preoperative* testing are listed in Chapter 10. Although there are many other situations in which pulmonary function testing is indicated, for reasons that are unclear, these tests are underutilized. This chapter describes instances in which testing is warranted and includes the basic tests to be ordered. Depending on the initial test results, additional studies may be indicated.

13A. THE SMOKER

Even if smokers have minimal respiratory symptoms, they should be tested by age 40. Depending on the results and a patient's smoking habits, repeat testing every 3 to 5 years is reasonable. The logic for early testing is shown in Figure 13-1. This shows the typical pattern of development of chronic obstructive pulmonary disease (COPD). Spirometry is the first test to have abnormal results. The innocuous cigarette cough may indicate significant airway obstruction. When confronted with an abnormal test result, a patient can often be convinced to make a serious attempt to stop smoking, which is a most important step to improving health. Figure 13-2 shows the average rates of decline in function in smokers and nonsmokers. The earlier the rapid loss of function can be interrupted in the smoker, the greater will be the life expectancy.

Test: Spirometry before and after bronchodilator

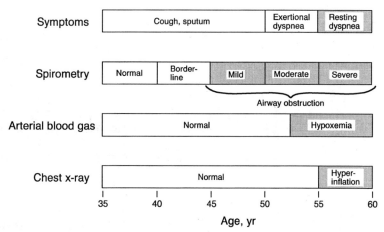

FIG. 13-1.   Progression of symptoms in chronic obstructive pulmonary disease (COPD) reflected by spirometry, arterial blood gas studies, and chest radiographs as a function of age in a typical case. Spirometry can detect COPD years before significant dyspnea occurs. (From PL Enright, RE Hyatt [eds]. *Office Spirometry: A Practical Guide to the Selection and Use of Spirometers.* Philadelphia: Lea & Febiger, 1987. By permission of Mayo Foundation.)

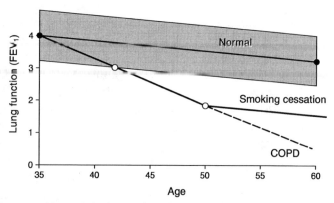

FIG. 13-2.   Normal decline in forced expiratory volume in 1 second (FEV$_1$) with age contrasted with the accelerated decline in COPD. Smoking cessation can halt this rapid decline. (From PL Enright, RE Hyatt [eds]. *Office Spirometry: A Practical Guide to the Selection and Use of Spirometers.* Philadelphia: Lea & Febiger, 1987. By permission of Mayo Foundation.)

13B. CHRONIC OBSTRUCTIVE PULMONARY DISEASE

Even if the clinical diagnosis of COPD is clear-cut, it is important to quantify the degree of impairment of pulmonary function. A forced expiratory volume in 1 second (FEV_1) of 50% of predicted portends future disabling disease. An FEV_1 of less than 800 mL predicts future carbon dioxide retention (respiratory insufficiency).

Repeating spirometry every 1 to 2 years establishes the rate of decline of values such as the FEV_1. The FEV_1 declines an average of 60 mL/yr in persons with COPD, compared with 25 to 30 mL/yr in normal subjects. An excessive rate of decline may indicate an asthmatic component that could benefit from inhaled steroids.

Tests: 1. Initially, spirometry before and after bronchodilator and determination of the diffusing capacity of carbon monoxide (DL_{CO}). Arterial blood gas studies are recommended when the FEV_1 is less than 50% predicted

2. Initially, if available, static lung volumes such as total lung capacity (TLC) and residual volume (RV)

3. Follow-up testing with spirometry is usually adequate

13C. ASTHMA

It is important to be sure that the patient with apparent asthma really has this disease. Remember that "not all that wheezes is asthma." Major airway lesions can cause stridor or wheezing, which has been mistaken for asthma. The flow-volume loop often identifies such lesions (see section 2K, page 19).

Testing is also important in patients with asthma in remission or with minimal symptoms. This provides a baseline against which to compare results of function tests during an attack and thus quantify the severity of the episode.

The patient should be taught to use a peak flowmeter. He or she should establish a baseline of peak expiratory flows when asthma is in remission by measuring flows each morning and evening before taking any treatment. Then the patient should continue to measure and record peak flows on a daily basis.

PEARL: It is crucial that the patients be taught to use a peak flowmeter correctly. They must take a *maximal* inhalation, place their lips around the mouthpiece (a nose clip is not needed), and give a *short, hard blast*. They should avoid making a full exhalation; the exhalation should mimic the quick exhalation used to blow out candles on a cake.

Having the patient with asthma monitor his or her pulmonary status is extremely important. An exacerbation is usually preceded by a gradual decline in peak flow, which the patient may not perceive. By the time the patient becomes symptomatic and dyspneic, flows may have greatly deteriorated. A decrease of about 20% from the symptom-free, baseline peak flow usually means treatments should be reinstated or increased and the physician contacted. It should be impressed on the patient and family that asthma is a serious, *potentially fatal* disease and that it must be respected and appropriately monitored and treated. Marked airway hyperresponsiveness and highly variable function are harbingers of severe attacks.

Tests: 1. Initial evaluation includes spirometry before and after bronchodilator—determination of $D_{L_{CO}}$ is optional. If there is any question about the diagnosis, a methacholine challenge study should be done (see Chapter 5)

2. For monitoring on a daily basis, a peak flowmeter is used

3. Periodic (annual) monitoring with spirometry and bronchodilator (more often in severe cases)

13D. ALLERGIC RHINITIS

Allergic rhinitis is often associated with asymptomatic hyperreactive airways. It may evolve into asthma. Thus, establishing a subject's baseline function and airway reactivity is justified.

Tests: Spirometry before and after bronchodilator. If the bronchodilator response is normal but concerns still exist, a methacholine challenge study (see Chapter 5) is indicated

13E. CHEST RADIOGRAPH WITH DIFFUSE INTERSTITIAL OR ALVEOLAR PATTERN

Several disorders can present with these patterns (see Table 12-2, page 113). Pulmonary function tests are performed to answer the following questions: Are the lung volumes decreased and, if so, by how much? Is the diffusing capacity reduced? Is there arterial oxygen desaturation at rest or with exercise? Not infrequently, oxygen saturation is normal at rest but decreases during exercise. The tests are also used to follow the course of the disease and the response to therapy.

Tests: 1. Spirometry before and after bronchodilator, determination of $D_{L_{CO}}$, and pulse oximetry at rest and during exercise. The bronchodilator is used because a subject with inherent hyperreactive airways might develop one of these disorders

2. Static lung volumes (such as TLC and RV) and lung compliance and recoil pressure at TLC (if available)

> **PEARL:** Rarely, an interstitial or alveolar pattern is associated with an increased $D_{L_{CO}}$. This can occur with intra-alveolar hemorrhage, such as in idiopathic hemosiderosis (Goodpasture's syndrome), in which hemoglobin in the alveoli binds to carbon monoxide. The $D_{L_{CO}}$ will decrease as the process improves.

13F. EXERTIONAL DYSPNEA

In *almost every case* of exertional dyspnea, pulmonary function tests should be performed. This approach applies even if the major abnormality appears to be nonpulmonary. We have seen patients with dyspnea who have received elaborate, and expensive, cardiovascular studies before pulmonary function studies were done, and the lungs proved to be the cause of the dyspnea. Also exercise-induced bronchospasm, often associated with inhalation of cold air, can be a cause of exertional dyspnea.

Tests: Spirometry before and after dilators and $D_{L_{CO}}$ testing. Determination of oxygen saturation at rest and exercise may be appropriate. For evaluation of exercise-induced bronchospasm, a methacholine challenge test should be done. In difficult cases, cardiopulmonary exercise testing may be helpful (see page 107)

13G. CHEST TIGHTNESS

Is the tightness caused by angina or episodic bronchospasm? The distinction is not always easy. Dyspnea is often associated with either disorder. If there is doubt, testing lung function, in addition to cardiac evaluation, is warranted.

Tests: Spirometry before and after bronchodilator. Methacholine challenge testing is done if bronchospasm remains a distinct possibility

13H. UNEXPLAINED CHRONIC COUGH

Some patients have cough that is not related to chronic bronchitis, bronchiectasis, or a current viral infection. The cough is usually nonproductive. The most frequent causes are listed in Table 13-1. Obviously, many causes are nonpulmonary. Those in which pulmonary function testing can be helpful are asthma, congestive heart failure, diffuse interstitial disease, and tracheal tumors.

Tests: Spirometry before and after bronchodilator, $D_{L_{CO}}$ test, methacholine challenge. A flow-volume loop also should be considered

> **PEARL:** In patients whose cough follows a viral tracheitis, systemic or inhaled steroids may provide relief, presumably by decreasing smoldering inflammation that is stimulating cough receptors.

13I. CORONARY ARTERY DISEASE

Because most patients with coronary artery disease (CAD) have been smokers, they have an increased risk of also having COPD. A strong case can be made for testing all such patients to assess their

TABLE 13-1.   Frequent causes of chronic cough

Postnasal drip
Asthma
Gastroesophageal reflux
Congestive heart failure
Diffuse interstitial disease
Postviral tracheitis
Angiotensin-converting enzyme inhibitor use
Bronchogenic carcinoma
Miscellaneous
   Tracheal tumors
   Temporal arteritis
   Oculopharyngeal muscular dystrophy
   Ulcerative colitis, Crohn's disease
   Foreign body

lung function. And, as noted in section 12H (page 114), congestive heart failure itself can impair lung function.

Test: Spirometry before and after bronchodilator

> **PEARL:** In addition to patients with CAD, those with hypertension may need to be tested, especially if therapy with β-adrenergic blockers is planned. These are usually contraindicated in COPD.

13J. RECURRENT BRONCHITIS OR PNEUMONIA

Not infrequently, asthma is mistaken for recurrent attacks of bronchitis. This mistake can be avoided by appropriate pulmonary function testing.

A subset of patients have recurrent bouts of pneumonia presenting as small pulmonary infiltrates. We have seen several such patients in whom the basic problem was occult asthma. Presumably the bronchoconstriction interfered with mucociliary clearance, thus predisposing to pneumonia. Regular use of inhaled steroids and β-agonists led to correction of the problem.

Tests: Spirometry before and after bronchodilator. Methacholine challenge testing is performed if bronchospasm remains a possibility

13K. NEUROMUSCULAR DISEASE

There are two reasons for performing pulmonary function tests, including maximal respiratory pressure tests, in patients with neuromuscular disease. First, dyspnea frequently develops in such patients, and it is important to establish the pathogenesis of the complaint. It might be pulmonary or cardiac in origin. Pulmonary function tests help to answer the question. Second, the tests can be useful for following the course of the disease.

Tests: Spirometry before and after dilator, DL_{CO} test, and determination of maximal respiratory pressures

13L. OCCUPATIONAL AND ENVIRONMENTAL EXPOSURES

Table 13-2 lists substances and occupations that can produce pulmonary abnormalities reflected in abnormal results of pulmonary

TABLE 13-2. Occupational and environmental exposures that can lead to pulmonary conditions

Industrial dusts
  Coal dust (coal workers' pneumoconiosis)
  Asbestos (asbestosis, pleural plaques, pleural effusion)
  Silica, quartz (silicosis)
  Cotton dust (byssinosis)
  Beryllium (berylliosis)
  Talc (talcosis)
Occupational asthma
  Plastics
  Isocyanates
  Animal dander, urine, feces
  Enzyme dusts
  Tea and coffee dust
  Grain dust
  Polyvinyl chloride (PVC) fumes
  Western red cedar—wood dusts
Hypersensitivity pneumonitis
  Farmer's lung
  Bird-fancier's disease
  Mushroom workers, other moldy dusts
  Humidifiers

tests. Some farsighted industries are monitoring workers' pulmonary function on a regular basis. This testing protects both the worker and the employer.

Tests: Spirometry before and after dilator

13M. SYSTEMIC DISEASES

Several nonpulmonary conditions are frequently associated with altered pulmonary function. Some of the more common ones are listed below, followed by the commonly abnormal pulmonary function test result(s).

1. Rheumatoid arthritis: DL_{CO} reduction is often the first change. Vital capacity may also be reduced, and airflow obstruction occurs in a few cases.
2. Scleroderma (systemic sclerosis): Reduced DL_{CO} is the first change, caused by minimal fibrosis often not visible by radiography. Later, lung volumes can decrease.
3. Systemic lupus erythematosus: Early decrease in DL_{CO}. Later, volumes may decrease dramatically, producing a

"vanishing lung," which may be more related to respiratory muscle weakness than to pulmonary fibrosis.

4. Wegener's granulomatosis: Both restrictive and obstructive patterns may be found, as well as major airway lesions.
5. Dermatomyositis: Muscle weakness and decreased $D_{L_{CO}}$ often occur.
6. Cirrhosis of the liver: In some cases, arterial oxygen desaturation is found. This is due to the development of arteriovenous shunts in the lungs or mediastinum. In many cases, the saturation is lower when the subject is standing (rather than lying), so-called orthodeoxia.
7. Relapsing polychondritis: Inflammatory degeneration of tracheal and bronchial cartilage can lead to a significant reduction in expiratory flows, an obstructive pattern.
8. Sjögren's syndrome: As many as half of affected patients have airway obstruction resistant to bronchodilators.

14

Approaches to Interpreting Pulmonary Function Tests

Different experts follow different approaches to pulmonary function interpretation. There is no universally accepted standard for interpretation, but the two most commonly cited standards are the 1986 American Thoracic Society Disability Standard [1] and the 1991 statement of the American Thoracic Society [2].

This chapter describes three approaches. The first uses the flow-volume curve and the normal predicted values. The second uses the test data without the flow-volume curve. The third uses a pulmonary function test "crib sheet" developed in the Mayo Clinic Division of Pulmonary and Critical Care Medicine and Internal Medicine as an instructional tool for residents and fellows.

14A. FLOW-VOLUME CURVE AVAILABLE

Step I

Examine the *flow-volume curve*. Is there any ventilatory limitation (that is, any loss of area)? If not, the test result is most likely normal.

1. Is the forced vital capacity (FVC) *normal*? If so, any significant restriction is essentially ruled out.
2. Is the FVC *reduced*? If so, either obstruction or restriction could be the cause (see Fig. 2-3, page 10).

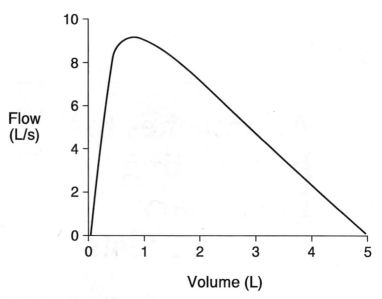

FIG. 14-1. Normal flow-volume curve.

3. Examine the contour of the flow-volume curve.
    a. Is it normal-appearing (Fig. 14-1)? If so, and if the FVC is
        normal, the test result is almost always normal. Proceed to
        steps V, VI, and VII. If the FVC is reduced and the flow-
        volume slope and ratio of forced expiratory volume in 1
        second to FVC (FEV$_1$/FVC ratio) are normal, restriction,
        occult asthma, or a nonspecific abnormality may be present
        (see section 2F, page 13, and section 3E, page 35). The total
        lung capacity (TLC) will have to be measured to make the
        differentiation.
    b. Is the curve scooped out with reduced flow-volume
        slope and low flows (Fig. 14-2)? An obstructive defect is
        most likely. Remember the occasional mixed restrictive-
        obstructive disorder.
4. Is the slope of the flow-volume curve increased (Fig. 14-3)?
    This finding is consistent with a pulmonary parenchymal
    restrictive process. The FVC, TLC, and diffusing capac-
    ity of carbon monoxide (D$_{L_{CO}}$) must be reduced to be
    certain.
5. If there is a flow-volume loop, is there any suggestion of a
    major airway lesion (Fig. 14-4)?

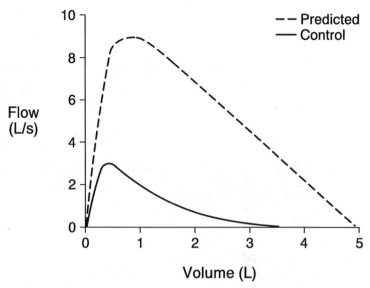

FIG. 14-2. Flow-volume curve in severe chronic obstructive pulmonary disease.

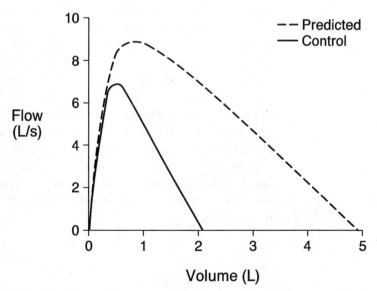

FIG. 14-3. Flow-volume curve in pulmonary fibrosis. Note steep slope and decreased volume.

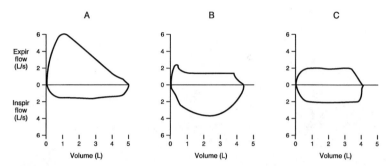

FIG. 14-4. Typical flow-volume curves associated with lesions of the major airway (carina to mouth). **A.** Typical variable extrathoracic lesion. **B.** Variable intrathoracic lesion. **C.** Fixed lesion.

Step II

Examine the *FEV₁ value.*

1. Is it *normal?* If so, all but borderline obstruction or restriction is ruled out. There are exceptions, namely, the rare variable extrathoracic lesion in which the FEV_1 can be normal but the maximal voluntary ventilation (MVV) is reduced because of inspiratory obstruction (as in Fig. 14-4A). Also subjects with respiratory muscle weakness (see section 9D, page 97) can initially present with dyspnea and a normal FEV_1.
2. Is the FEV_1 *reduced* by more than 15 to 20%? If so, the decrease is most often due to airway obstruction. It could be caused by a restrictive process, however, and thus, the FEV_1/FVC ratio needs to be evaluated. Nevertheless, if the TLC value is available, check it first. An increase in TLC by more than 15 to 20% favors obstructive disease. A normal or increased value excludes a pulmonary restrictive process by definition. A normal TLC can occur in the rare mixed obstructive-restrictive disorder. A reduced TLC is expected with a restrictive process.

Step III

Examine the *FEV₁/FVC ratio.*

1. If the absolute ratio is *decreased* to 75% or less, an obstructive process is present, except in the elderly, in whom the lower limit of normal is about 65%.

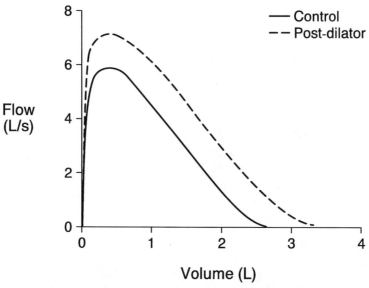

FIG. 14-5. Control curve shows mild reduction in forced vital capacity (FVC) and forced expiratory volume in 1 second (FEV_1) and a normal FEV_1/FVC ratio. After administration of a bronchodilator, the flow-volume curve (dashed line) shows a parallel shift to the right with an increase in FVC and FEV_1 but no change in the FEV_1/FVC ratio. The patient has occult asthma.

2. If the ratio is *normal*, an obstructive process is usually excluded. An exception is the case of nonspecific ventilatory limitation, in which the FVC and FEV_1 are reduced and the FEV_1/FVC ratio, flow-volume slope, and TLC are all normal (see section 3E, page 35). Administration of a bronchodilator often exposes occult asthma (Fig. 14-5), but occasionally a methacholine challenge test is needed. Airway resistance, if available, is often increased and can be helpful in identifying the patient with occult asthma.

3. The ratio is *normal* or *increased* with a pure restrictive disorder. Patients with a reduced FVC, reduced FEV_1, normal to increased FEV_1/FVC ratio, and normal response to bronchodilator usually have a restrictive process. If there is doubt, have the TLC or DL_{CO} measured; they should be low. If the TLC test is not available, check the chest radiograph for evidence of reduction in TLC, or estimate TLC by the radiographic technique discussed in section 3C (page 31).

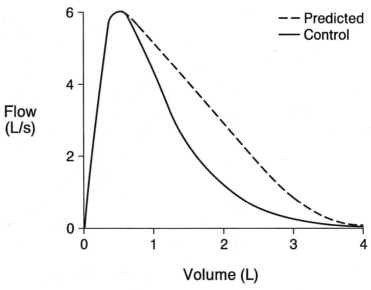

FIG. 14-6.   The unusual flow-volume curve in which the forced expiratory volume in 1 second is normal but the forced expiratory flow rate over the middle 50% of the forced vital capacity is reduced. Note that the peak flow is normal but the lower 70% is very scooped out.

Step IV

Examine the *expiratory flow values*.

1. The forced expiratory flow rate over the middle 50% of the FVC (FEF_{25-75}) almost always changes in the same direction as the FEV_1. This test may be more sensitive for detecting early airway obstruction. The FEF_{25-75} is occasionally reduced in the face of a normal FVC, FEV_1, and MVV. The flow-volume curve has a characteristic appearance. This result tends to occur in elderly persons with minimal symptoms (Fig. 14-6). Also see section 7A (page 75).
2. $FEF_{25,50,75}$. These flows change directionally in concert with the FEV_1 and FEF_{25-75}.

Step V

Examine the *MVV*.

1. The MVV will change in most cases in a manner similar to that of the FEV_1. With a *normal* FEV_1, a normal MVV should be

expected (FEV$_1$ × 40 = predicted MVV). Consider the lower limit to be FEV$_1$ × 30.

2. If the FEV$_1$ is *reduced* by *obstructive* disease, the MVV will also be reduced. However, the rule that FEV$_1$ × 40 = MVV is not always true in obstructive disease.

3. If the FEV$_1$ is *reduced* by a *restrictive* process, the MVV usually is reduced, but not always as much as suggested by the FEV$_1$ (some subjects with a very steep flow-volume curve can have normal flows high in the vital capacity; see Fig. 2-4 *D*, page 12).

4. If the FEV$_1$ is *normal* but the MVV is *reduced* below the lower limit, consider the following possibilities:

   a. Poor patient performance due to weakness, lack of coordination, fatigue, coughing induced by the maneuver, or unwillingness to give maximal effort (best judged by the technician).

   b. Does the patient have a neuromuscular disorder? The MVV is usually the first routine test to have an abnormal result. Consider ordering maximal respiratory pressure tests (see Chapter 9).

   c. Does the subject have a major airway lesion? The MVV is reduced in all three types of lesions shown in Figure 14-4; to evaluate this, the flow-volume loop needs to be evaluated.

   d. Is the subject massively obese? The MVV tends to decrease before the FEV$_1$ does.

Step VI

Examine the response to *bronchodilator*.

1. Is the response *normal* (0–10% increase in FEV$_1$)?

2. Is the response *increased* (FEV$_1$ increased by 12% and 200 mL)? If so, this finding suggests hyperreactive airways. A case of occult asthma may be exposed by such a response. (Remember the possible effect of effort on the FEV$_1$, section 5D, page 53, and Fig. 5-4, page 55.) However, the patient with asthma may not always have an increased response. The response can vary with the state of the disease.

Step VII

Examine the $D_{L_{CO}}$.

1. Is the $D_{L_{CO}}$ *normal*? This result is consistent with normal lungs. However, the $D_{L_{CO}}$ may also be normal in chronic

bronchitis, asthma, major airway lesions, extrapulmonary restriction, neuromuscular disease, and obesity.

2. Is the $D_{L_{CO}}$ *reduced*? This finding is characteristic of pulmonary parenchymal restrictive disorders. It is also consistent with anatomic emphysema and pulmonary vascular disorders. However, values can also be reduced in chronic bronchitis, asthma, and heart failure.

   An isolated reduction in the $D_{L_{CO}}$ (other tests within normal limits) should raise the possibility of pulmonary vascular disorders, such as scleroderma, primary pulmonary hypertension, recurrent emboli, and various vasculitides. Chemotherapeutic agents can also produce this finding.

3. Is the $D_{L_{CO}}$ *increased*? This result occurs in some patients with asthma and in some very obese subjects. Alveolar hemorrhage may also increase the $D_{L_{CO}}$, as can polycythemia vera, left-to-right intracardiac shunt, or any process that produces pulmonary vascular engorgement.

Step VIII

Examine *other test results* that you may have available. They should confirm the interpretation at which you have already arrived and fit the patterns in Table 12-1, pages 110 and 111.

14B. FLOW-VOLUME CURVE NOT AVAILABLE

Step I

Examine the *FVC*.

1. Is it *normal*? If so, any significant restriction is ruled out.
2. Is it *reduced*? If so, this finding could be due to either obstruction or restriction (see Fig. 2-3, page 10).

Step II

Examine the *FEV₁*.

1. Is it *normal*? If so, any significant obstruction or restriction is ruled out. There are exceptions, namely, the rare variable extrathoracic lesion in which the FEV_1 can be normal but the MVV is reduced because of the inspiratory obstruction. Also, subjects with respiratory muscle weakness can initially present with dyspnea and a normal FEV_1.

2. Is it *reduced* by more than 15 to 20%? If so, this finding is most often due to airway obstruction. However, it could be caused by a restrictive process, and thus the FEV_1/FVC ratio needs to be evaluated. First, though, if the TLC is available, it should be checked. A TLC that is increased more than 15% favors obstruction. By definition, a normal or increased TLC rules out pure parenchymal restriction. The TLC is occasionally normal in a mixed obstructive-restrictive disorder. A reduced TLC is expected in a pure restrictive process.

Step III

Examine the *FEV_1/FVC*.

1. If the absolute ratio is *decreased* to 75% or less, an obstructive process is present. The lower limit of normal in the elderly is approximately 65%.

2. If the ratio is *normal,* this finding excludes the usual obstructive process. An exception is nonspecific ventilatory limitation, in which the FVC and FEV_1 are reduced and the FEV_1/FVC ratio and TLC are normal (see section 3E, page 35). Administration of a bronchodilator usually exposes occult asthma, but occasionally a methacholine challenge test is needed.

3. Otherwise, the ratio is normal or increased in a pure restrictive process. A reduced FVC, reduced FEV_1, normal to increased FEV_1/FVC ratio, and normal response to bronchodilator usually indicate a restrictive defect. If there is any doubt, the TLC or $D_{L_{CO}}$ should be measured; they should be low. If the TLC is not available, the chest radiograph can be checked for evidence of reduction in the TLC, or the TLC can be estimated by the radiographic technique described in section 3C, page 31.

Step IV

Examine the *expiratory flow values.*

1. The *FEF_{25-75}* almost invariably changes in the same direction as the FEV_1. This test may be more sensitive than the FEV_1 for detecting early airway disease.

2. Rarely, the FEF_{25-75} is reduced in the face of a normal FVC, FEV_1, and MVV. This situation tends to occur

in elderly persons who have few symptoms (see section 7A, page 75).

Step V

Examine the *MVV*.

1. The MVV will, in most cases, change in a manner similar to that of the FEV_1. With a normal FEV_1, a normal MVV should be expected (that is, $FEV_1 \times 40$ = predicted MVV). Consider the lower limit to be $FEV_1 \times 30$.
2. If the FEV_1 is *reduced* by *obstructive* disease, the MVV will also be reduced. However, the rule that $FEV_1 \times 40$ = MVV is not always true in obstructive disease.
3. If the FEV_1 is *reduced* by a *restrictive* process, the MVV usually is reduced. However, the MVV is not always reduced as much as suggested by the reduction in FEV_1 because some subjects with a restrictive process have normal flows high in the vital capacity.
4. If the FEV_1 is *normal* but the MVV is *reduced*, consider the following possibilities:
   a. The patient's performance was poor because of weakness, lack of coordination, fatigue, coughing induced by the maneuver, or unwillingness to give a maximal effort (best judged by the technician).
   b. Does the patient have a neuromuscular disorder? The MVV test is usually the first routine test to have an abnormal result. Determination of maximal respiratory pressures should be considered (see Chapter 9).
   c. Does the patient have a major airway lesion? The MVV is reduced in all three types of lesions (see Fig. 2-7, page 18).
   d. Is the subject massively obese? The MVV tends to decrease before the FEV_1 does.

Step VI

Examine the response to *bronchodilator*.

1. Is the response *normal* (that is, 0–10% increase in the FEV_1)?
2. Is the response *increased* (FEV_1 increased by 12% and 200 mL)? If so, this finding suggests hyperreactive airways.

A case of occult asthma may be exposed by such a response. (The possible effect of effort on the FEV_1 needs to be considered; see section 5D, page 53.) However, the patient with asthma may not always have an increased response. It can vary with the state of the disease.

Step VII

Examine the D_{LCO}.

1. Is the D_{LCO} *normal*? This finding is consistent with normal lungs. However, the D_{LCO} may also be normal in chronic bronchitis, asthma, major airway lesions, extrapulmonary restriction, neuromuscular disease, and obesity.

2. Is the D_{LCO} *reduced*? This finding is characteristic of pulmonary restrictive disorders. It is also consistent with anatomic emphysema and pulmonary vascular disease. However, values can also be reduced in chronic bronchitis, asthma, chronic obstructive pulmonary disease, and heart failure.

   An isolated reduction in the D_{LCO} (other test results are within normal limits) should raise the possibility of pulmonary vascular disorders such as scleroderma, primary pulmonary hypertension, recurrent emboli, and various vasculitides.

3. Is the D_{LCO} *increased*? This finding occurs in some patients with asthma and in some very obese subjects. Alveolar hemorrhage may also increase the D_{LCO}, as can polycythemia vera, left-to-right intracardiac shunt, or any process that produces pulmonary vascular engorgement.

Step VIII

Examine *other test results* that may be available. They should confirm the interpretation already arrived at and fit the patterns given in Table 12-1, pages 110 and 111.

14C. PULMONARY FUNCTION TEST CRIB SHEET

This summary was developed for use by internal medicine residents and pulmonary fellows at Mayo Clinic. It is self-explanatory.

Spirometry Interpretation

Look at the FVC and the FEV_1/FVC ratio:

1. Does the curve suggest obstruction (scooped out), restriction (shaped like a witch's hat), or a special case (see below)?
2. Is the FEV_1/FVC ratio reduced (<70% or lower limit of normal), indicating obstruction?

If the FEV_1/FVC ratio is less than 70% → *obstruction algorithm*

FEV_1 >80% Borderline
<80% Mild
<60% Moderate
<40% Severe

REMEMBER: Obstruction, 80/60/40

If the FEV_1/FVC ratio is normal → *restriction algorithm*

FVC >80% Normal
<80% Mild
<60% Moderate
<50% Severe

REMEMBER: Restriction, 80/60/50

(Caution: In some cases the FEV_1/FVC ratio is normal but obstruction is present. See "Nonspecific Pattern," below. A bronchodilator response, increased airways resistance, or a positive methacholine challenge test can be helpful in some of these cases.)

Bronchodilator response is positive if FEV_1 increases >12% *and* >200 mL.

A large bronchodilator response is predictive of:
More rapid decrease in lung function
More severe exacerbations
Increased risk for rapid decline and death

Flow-Volume Curve

1. Gives clues about the presence of obstruction or restriction (see Fig. 2-5, 2-7B and C)
2. Is the best indicator of test quality (see Fig. 2-6):

The curve should be examined for maneuver errors, including the following: B) slow start, C&D) poor blast, E) early termination, F&G) cough or interruption in the first second

3.   Gives clues about unusual conditions, such as the following:

Plateau on curve may indicate a central airway obstructive process (Fig. 2-7F)

Normal variant curve (tracheal plateau) common in young adults, especially women (Fig. 2-6H)

Inspiratory obstruction with variable extrathoracic obstruction (Fig. 2-7D) (e.g., goiter, tracheal tumor, subglottic stenosis, rheumatoid arthritis with cricoarytenoid fusion)

Expiratory obstruction with variable intrathoracic (tracheal) obstruction (Fig. 2-7E)

A convex flow-volume curve (Fig. 2-6D) may be found in the following:

Children

Neuromuscular weakness (see below)

Poor performance

Methacholine Challenge

This is positive if >20% decrease in FEV_1 after 25 mg/mL. Elements needed for asthma diagnosis: (1) evidence of airway hyperresponsiveness, (2) obstruction varying over time, (3) evidence of airway inflammation.

Lung Volumes

Gas-dilution techniques (He dilution or N_2 washout) underestimate lung volumes in obstructive disorders compared with plethysmography

Obstructive disorders have a TLC that is high (hyperinflation) or normal

An increased RV (air trapping) and an increased RV/TLC ratio

Restrictive disorders generally have a low TLC

RV may be high (muscular restriction, chest wall limitation, superimposed obstruction)

Neuromuscular Restriction

This looks like pulmonary restriction in spirometry, but:

Lung volumes usually show decreased TLC, increased RV

FVC is *disproportionately* reduced relative to TLC (quantify severity based on FVC, not TLC)

RV/TLC is *increased* (obstruction is not the only cause of high RV/TLC)

Maximal respiratory pressures are reduced

Flow-volume curve looks like poor performance or a child's curve

Early in the course of disorders causing muscular weakness (e.g., amyotrophic lateral sclerosis), maximal respiratory pressures may be reduced, but vital capacity, FEV_1, and MVV are still normal

Nonspecific Pattern (not defined in the literature)

Some patients have a low FEV_1 and FVC, normal FEV_1/FVC ratio, and normal TLC. In laboratories with a body plethysmograph, this can be further evaluated with measurement of airways resistance (Raw). If it is increased, we consider it an obstructive disorder and grade severity based on FEV_1. If Raw is normal, we call it a nonspecific pattern (see section 2F, page 13 and page 37). The most common associated clinical conditions are asthma, obesity, congestive heart failure, and chest wall-limiting conditions. An alternative or additional option is to perform methacholine challenge because airways hyperresponsiveness is often associated.

D_{LCO}

This is *reduced* in patients with a gas exchange abnormality (e.g., emphysema, idiopathic pulmonary fibrosis, other parenchymal or vascular processes).

A low D_{LCO} is characteristic of emphysema (not as sensitive or specific as high-resolution computed tomography), whereas in asthma and some cases of obstructive chronic bronchitis D_{LCO} is normal.

D_{LCO} may be reduced in pulmonary hypertension, but is insensitive for detecting cases.

D_{LCO} is often used to monitor for adverse pulmonary effect of chemotherapy.

Be sure to use D_{LCO} adjusted for low hemoglobin for such patients.

D_{LCO} may be *increased* in: (1) asthma, (2) obesity, (3) left-to-right shunt, (4) polycythemia, (5) hyperdynamic states, postexercise, (6) pulmonary hemorrhage, (7) supine position.

Maximal Respiratory Pressures ("Bugles")

These are used to assess respiratory muscle strength. If low, they indicate *muscle weakness or poor performance*. Inspiratory pressure is mostly a function of diaphragmatic strength. Tetraplegics show reduced expiratory pressures with inspiratory pressures (diaphragm) relatively preserved. Diaphragmatic paralysis is the opposite.

Obesity

Obesity has a small but significant effect on pulmonary function. The increased chest wall impedance causes a restrictive pattern in some obese patients. On average, a person with a body mass index of 35 will have a 5 to 10% reduction in FVC. TLC is usually not reduced to the same degree as FVC. Obstruction is not caused by obesity. Obese people may wheeze because they breathe near residual volume, sometimes called "pseudo-asthma." $D_{L_{CO}}$ is normal or increased.

REFERENCES

1. American Thoracic Society. Evaluation of impairment/disability secondary to respiratory disorders. *Am Rev Respir Dis* 133:1205–1209, 1986.
2. American Thoracic Society. Lung function testing: Selection of reference values and interpretative strategies. *Am Rev Respir Dis* 144:1202–1218, 1991.

15

Illustrative Cases

The cases presented in this chapter demonstrate many of the points made in the preceding text. A few examples are of unusual cases, but most present problems that are commonly evaluated in the pulmonary function laboratory.

For most of the cases, the flow-volume curve should be studied first. After a preliminary interpretation is reached, the measurements should be reviewed to determine whether they support or change this interpretation. Frequently, some questions are posed, and an attempt should be made to answer them before the answers are read. (The cases are not arranged in a particular order. In the tables, abnormal values are indicated by an asterisk [*]. The types of cases are listed on pages 227 and 228. Also, the abbreviations used in the chapter are defined on pages xi–xiii.)

CASE 1

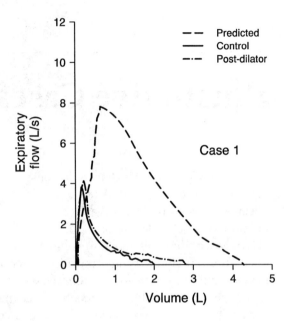

71 y   M   Wt 195 lb (88 kg)   Ht 69 in. (175 cm)

	Normal	Observed	% predicted	Post-dilator
Spirometry				
FVC (L)	4.29	1.94*	45	2.76
FEV$_1$ (L)	3.29	1.03*	31	1.25
FEV$_1$/FVC (%)	77	53*		
FEF$_{25-75}$ (L/s)	2.8	0.4*	15	0.5
MVV (L/min)	125	51*	41	
Volumes				
TLC (L)	6.61	9.37*	142	
RV/TLC (%)	35	75*	214	
D$_{L_{CO}}$ (mL/min/mm Hg)	25	10*	40	

Comments and Questions

This patient had a smoking history of 74 pack-years and was still smoking. He complained of progressive breathlessness and wheezing on mild exertion. He had a family history of pulmonary disease.

1. How would you interpret this test?
2. Can you make a statement as to the patient's underlying lung disease?
3. Does the reduced $D_{L_{CO}}$ suggest anything?

CASE 1

Answers

1. The patient has severe ventilatory limitation on an obstructive basis. Significant hyperinflation is present with an increased TLC and RV/TLC ratio. There is a small but significant response to bronchodilator. The reduced diffusing capacity suggests the presence of anatomic emphysema.

2. If only the results of spirometry were available, it could be said that "there is severe ventilatory limitation on an obstructive basis, but a small restrictive component cannot be ruled out without a measurement of total lung capacity." Of course, if a chest radiograph showed hyperinflation, then it is almost certain that the abnormalities were all obstructive.

3. In this case with the hyperinflation and obstruction, the low D_{LCO} is consistent with anatomic emphysema, and high-resolution computed tomography would be expected to confirm this. In case 10 (page 163), in which the TLC is very low and the slope of the flow-volume curve is steep, the low D_{LCO} probably reflects the presence of some type of fibrosis. Often when the D_{LCO} is low, however, only a general statement can be made, such as "the low D_{LCO} suggests the presence of a parenchymal or vascular abnormality."

CASE 2

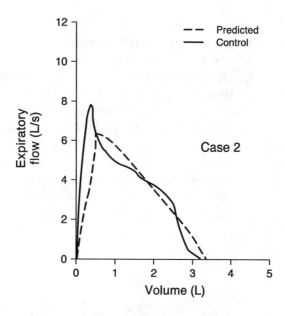

36 y   F   Wt 183 lb (83 kg)   Ht 64 in. (162 cm)

	Normal	Observed	% predicted	Post-dilator
Spirometry				
FVC (L)	3.69	3.27	89	3.36
FEV_1 (L)	3.10	2.93	94	2.93
FEV_1/FVC (%)	84	89		
FEF_{25-75} (L/s)	3.1	4.0	131	
MVV (L/min)	113	121	106	
Volumes				
TLC (L)	5.04	4.62	92	
RV/TLC (%)	27	21	78	
DL_{CO} (mL/min/mm Hg)	24	24	100	

Questions

1. Does the patient have ventilatory limitation?
2. Do the test values support your impression?
3. Is the configuration of the flow-volume curve normal?

CASE 2

Answers

1. There is no ventilatory limitation.
2. The test values are all normal.
3. Over most of the vital capacity, flow decreases in a relatively gradual, steady fashion. However, at 2.4 L of expired volume, there is a "knee" in the curve after which flow decreases rapidly. This contour is not due to a major airway lesion but is a normal variant that is often found in nonsmokers, especially women. This patient had never smoked. This curve shape is due to the point of critical narrowing staying in the trachea until the "knee" is reached (see Fig. 2-6H, page 16). This is called a "tracheal plateau."

CASE 3

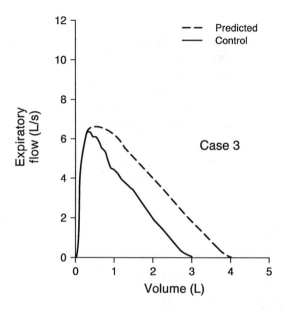

29 y   F   Wt 284 lb (129 kg)   Ht 65 in. (165 cm)

	Normal	*Observed*	*% predicted*
Spirometry			
FVC (L)	3.94	3.06*	78
FEV$_1$ (L)	3.34	2.64*	79
FEV$_1$/FVC (%)	85	86	
FEF$_{25-75}$ (L/s)	3.4	2.8	85
MVV (L/min)	120	90	75
Volumes			
TLC (L)	5.18	4.23	82
RV/TLC (%)	24	28	117
D$_{L_{CO}}$ (mL/min/mm Hg)	25	24	96

Questions

1. Is there any ventilatory limitation?
2. On the basis of the given data, what diagnosis would you give?
3. Is there anything unique about this patient?
4. The patient had been a light smoker since age 20 years, smoking an average of eight cigarettes a day, or 3.6 pack-years. She reported episodes of bronchitis with wheezing and breathlessness. Is there any other test you would order?

CASE 3

Answers

1. The control flow-volume curve shows some loss of area, consistent with a mild ventilatory limitation.
2. The low but normal TLC, the proportionate reduction in FVC and FEV_1, the normal FEV_1/FVC ratio, and the normal DL_{CO} indicate the presence of "nonspecific ventilatory limitation" (see section 3E, page 35).
3. The patient is obese; the BMI is 47.4 kg/m^2 (normal, <30).
4. On the basis of the history, a methacholine challenge test is a reasonable procedure to order because many patients with asthma are diagnosed as having bronchitis.

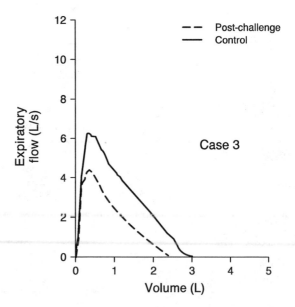

As shown in the figure, the patient has hyperreactive airways with a markedly reduced flow-volume curve after methacholine. The FEV_1 decreased 21%.

The diagnosis now becomes "mild ventilatory limitation due to asthma and probably obesity."

CASE 4

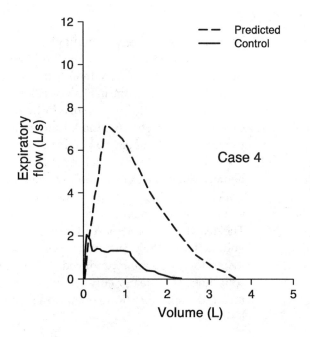

76 y   M   Wt 170 lb (77 kg)   Ht 66 in. (168 cm)

Spirometry	Normal	Observed	% predicted
FVC (L)	3.69	2.44*	66
FEV$_1$ (L)	2.83	1.33*	47
FEV$_1$/FVC (%)	77	55*	
FEF$_{25-75}$ (L/s)	2.6	0.7*	
MVV (L/min)	112	30*	27

Questions

1. What is your estimate of the degree of limitation?
2. What is causing the limitation?
3. Is there anything unusual about the test data?
4. Is there anything unusual about the flow-volume curve?
5. Is there any other test that you would order?

CASE 4

Answers

1. There is a severe degree of limitation.
2. On the basis of the test data, the limitation is obstructive.
3. The decrease in the MVV to 27% predicted is greater than might be expected from an FEV_1 of 47% predicted. This finding should suggest poor patient effort, a neuromuscular process, or a major airway lesion. In this case, the technicians thought the patient gave a good effort.
4. There is something unusual about the flow-volume curve; namely, there is a plateau in flow at about 1.3 L/s over the upper 50% of the FVC that is abnormal. It is characteristic of a major airway lesion.
5. The test that should be ordered is an inspiratory flow-volume loop. The expiratory curve and the corresponding inspiratory loop are reproduced in the figure below as the solid lines. The nearly equal reduction in maximal expiratory and inspiratory flows points to a relatively fixed airway lesion.

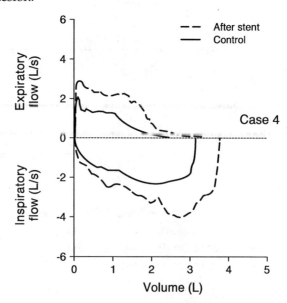

The patient was found to have Wegener's granulomatosis. Bronchoscopy revealed narrowing of both main stem bronchi and of several lobar bronchi. Ordinarily, single obstructing lesions below the carina cannot be detected with certainty. However, because both main stem bronchi were involved, a characteristic abnormality in the flow-volume loop could be detected.

With the patient under general anesthesia, the left main stem bronchus and bronchus intermedius were dilated, and stents were placed in both. The right main stem bronchus was also dilated. The dashed flow-volume loop in the figure above was obtained 1 month after this procedure, and although the flows are not normal, they are much improved.

CASE 5

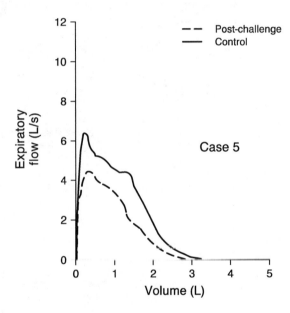

52 y   F   Wt 207 lb (94 kg)   Ht 63 in. (160 cm)

Spirometry	Normal	Observed	% predicted	Post-challenge
FVC (L)	3.17	3.37	106	
FEV$_1$ (L)	2.61	2.45	94	2.10 (−14%)
FEV$_1$/FVC (%)	83	73		
FEF$_{25-75}$ (L/s)	2.6	1.7	67	

Comments

This 52-year-old woman complained of chronic cough and mild dyspnea on exertion. She had never smoked. She was somewhat heavy for her height; the BMI is 36.7 kg/m^2.

The control flow-volume curve in the figure is normal and typical of a nonsmoker. Spirometry data are also normal, but the flow-volume curve shows increased curvature over the lower 50% of the FVC, suggesting mild airway obstruction.

The patient underwent a methacholine challenge study, and the FEV_1 decreased 14%, which is a negative test result. The post-challenge curve, selected because it had the largest FEV_1, is shown in the first figure.

The peak expiratory flow of the effort in the first figure is 4.5 L/s. Another post-challenge effort with a peak expiratory flow of 5.6 L/s was obtained, as shown below. This curve is curvilinear, consistent with airway obstruction. Because of the better effort reflected in the higher peak flow, this curve should have been selected. Its FEV_1 is 1.88 L, showing a 23% decrease and hence a positive result of methacholine challenge. This example confirms the statement in section 5D (page 53), namely, that a slightly submaximal effort can lead to an overestimation of the FEV_1.

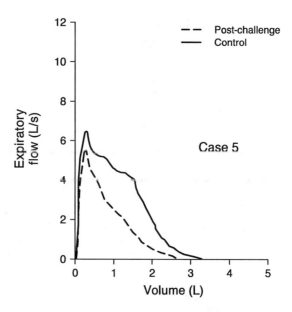

CASE 6

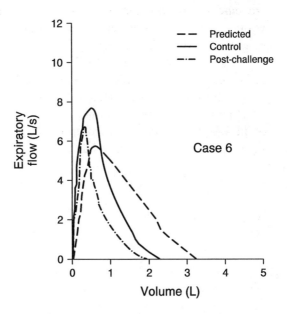

51 y F Wt 182 lb (83 kg) Ht 63 in. (160 cm)

	Normal	Observed	% predicted	Post-challenge
Spirometry				
FVC (L)	3.24	2.38*	73	1.98 (−17%)
FEV$_1$ (L)	2.67	1.96*	73	1.55 (−21%)
FEV$_1$/FVC (%)	82	83		78
FEF$_{25-75}$ (L/s)	2.6	2.1	80	
MVV (L/min)	101	83	82	
Volumes				
TLC (L)	4.9	4.06	83	
RV/TLC (%)	34	33	97	
D$_{CO}$ (mL/min/mm Hg)	22	21	95	

Comments

This 51-year-old woman had active rheumatoid arthritis and was receiving low-dose prednisone. She had never smoked. Because of a history of an allergic reaction to a medication that produced mild dyspnea and cough, a methacholine challenge test was ordered.

The control study fit our definition of mild "nonspecific ventilatory limitation" (see section 3E, page 35); that is, the TLC is within normal limits, the FEV$_1$ and FVC are both abnormally low, and the FEV_1/FVC ratio is normal. The normal DL_{CO} does not suggest any parenchymal problem, such as fibrosis, even though the flow-volume curve is rather steep. The patient is somewhat heavy for height; the BMI is 32.4 kg/m^2.

Despite the normal FEV_1/FVC ratio, the patient has hyperreactive airways with a 21% decrease in the FEV_1 associated with cough and some chest tightness. Thus, in this patient a "nonspecific" pattern is obscuring a mild case of asthma. There is a hint of increased curvature of the control flow-volume plot low in the vital capacity, but this is very subtle.

CASE 7

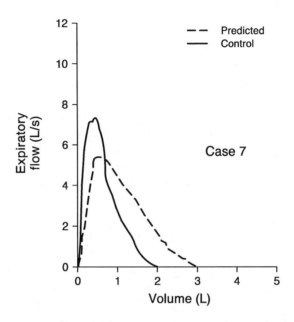

67 y   F   Wt 198 lb (90 kg)   Ht 64 in. (162 cm)

	Normal	*Observed*	*% predicted*
Spirometry			
FVC (L)	2.92	1.95*	67
FEV$_1$ (L)	2.33	1.68*	72
FEV$_1$/FVC (%)	80	86	
FEF$_{25-75}$ (L/s)	2.1	2.2	105
MVV (L/min)	90	64	71
Volumes			
TLC (L)	4.96	3.95	80
RV/TLC (%)	41	47	113
D$_{L_{CO}}$ (mL/min/mm Hg)	21	21	100

Comments and Questions

The patient is a nonsmoker and complains of shortness of breath at times while hurrying on a level surface. On occasion she has noted some wheezing.

1. Does the patient have ventilatory limitation? If so, on what basis?
2. Is there anything unusual about the patient?
3. Is there any additional study you would want?

CASE 7

Answers

1. The patient does have mild ventilatory limitation. This appears to be nonspecific, with equal reduction in the FEV_1 and FVC and thus a normal ratio. The low-normal TLC suggests a possible mild restrictive defect, as does the initial steep slope of the flow-volume curve. In addition, however, the increased curvature of the flow-volume curve raises the possibility of a mild airway obstruction. Thus, the limitation is likely due to a mixed restrictive-obstructive process.
2. The patient is somewhat heavy for her height; the BMI is 34.3 kg/m². This may contribute to the reduced FVC and low TLC.
3. With a history of wheezing in a nonsmoker, a methacholine challenge study is in order. The figure below shows a markedly positive result of methacholine challenge with a 41% decrease in the FEV_1. Despite this, the FEV_1/FVC ratio stayed in the high-normal range. The patient experienced some dyspnea, which was promptly relieved by an inhaled bronchodilator.

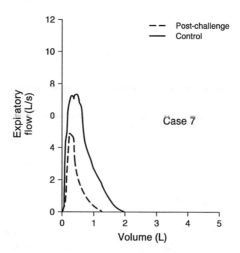

In summary, this is a case of obstructive airway disease (asthma) in which the FEV_1/FVC ratio was high-normal on presentation. Usually, this finding does not suggest airway obstruction. However, occult asthma can present with this picture. Also, the low-normal TLC does not suggest obstruction in most situations, but this case is an exception.

CASE 8

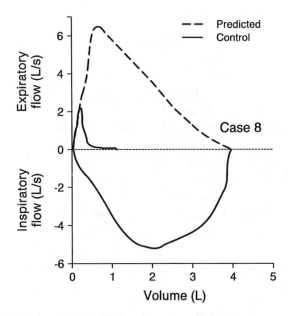

Case 8

43 y   F   Wt 134 lb (61 kg)   Ht 66 in. (168 cm)

	Normal	Observed	% predicted
Spirometry			
FVC (L)	3.71	1.22*	33
FEV$_1$ (L)	3.05	0.51*	17
FEV$_1$/FVC (%)	82	42*	
FEF$_{25-75}$ (L/s)	2.8	0.1*	
MVV (L/min)	111	40*	36
Volumes			
TLC (L)	5.34	6.07	114
RV/TLC (%)	31	32	103
D$_{L_{CO}}$ (mL/min/mm Hg)	24	23	

Comments and Questions

The inspiratory loop was obtained after a slow expiration to residual volume. This SVC was used to compute the RV/TLC ratio. This 43-year-old woman with a 16 pack-year smoking history had the recent onset of chest discomfort, shortness of breath, and wheezing after a viral-like illness, 3 weeks before this study.

1. What features of the control flow-volume loop are unusual?
2. Are any features of the function data unusual?
3. What might be the patient's problem?
4. Is there a procedure you might request?

CASE 8

Answers

1. The striking features of the control flow-volume loop are as follows:
   a. The marked reduction in expiratory flows with reasonably normal inspiratory flows—variable intrathoracic lesion
   b. The marked difference between the expiratory FVC (1.2 L) and the inspiratory vital capacity (4.0 L)
2. The spirometric values are typical of severe obstruction. The only possibly unusual finding is the normal DL_{CO} with this degree of obstruction, but this situation can occur.
3. The sudden onset of this degree of obstruction and the marked difference in the inspiratory and expiratory flows and volumes suggest a major airway lesion.
4. The appropriate procedure would be bronchoscopy.

The patient had an abnormal chest radiograph with hilar enlargement, and bronchoscopy revealed a large lesion almost occluding the intrathoracic trachea. The squamous cell lesion was managed initially with laser therapy; the symptoms and the second flow-volume loop improved. Thoracic radiation and chemotherapy led to disappearance of the tumor, and the third flow-volume loop was normal.

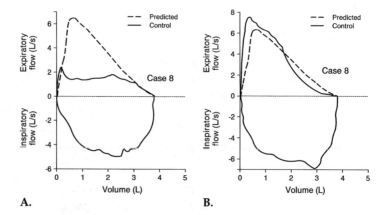

A.   B.

CASE 9

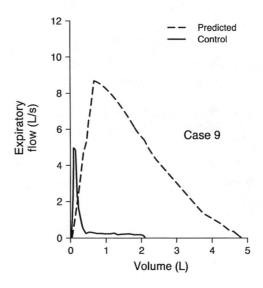

67 y   M   Wt 189 lb (86 kg)   Ht 71 in. (180 cm)

	Normal	*Observed*	*% predicted*	*Post-dilator*
Spirometry				
FVC (L)	4.79	2.06*	43	2.67
FEV$_1$ (L)	3.67	0.56*	15	0.75
FEV$_1$/FVC (%)	77	27*		
FEF$_{25-75}$ (L/s)	31	0.2*	6	
MVV (L/min)	136	29*	21	
Volumes				
TLC (L)	7.02	8.64*	123	
RV/TLC (%)	32	69*	216	
D$_{Lco}$ (mL/min/mm Hg)	27	21	79	

Comments and Questions

This 67-year-old man had a history of 59 pack-years of smoking. He had complained 5 years previously of shortness of breath while walking on a level surface. His dyspnea, often accompanied by wheezing, had become progressively worse, to the point that he had to stop walking after one block.

1. How would you describe the flow-volume curve?
2. Do the test results support your impression? (Incidentally, the post-dilator flow-volume curve is not shown for the sake of clarity, but it did show slightly higher flows and volumes.)

CASE 9

Answers

1. There is a significant loss of area under the flow-volume curve, and the curve is typical of obstruction. Thus, "severe ventilatory limitation secondary to airway obstruction" would be correct.

2. The increased TLC and RV are consistent with this interpretation, as are the markedly reduced FEV_1 and FEF_{25-75}.

The DL_{CO} is in the low-normal range, which argues against significant anatomic emphysema. This is a good example of a patient with chronic bronchitis who responds to a bronchodilator and has desaturation with exercise. Not shown was the oximetry result—a resting oxygen saturation of 94% that decreased to 86% with mild exercise.

CASE 10

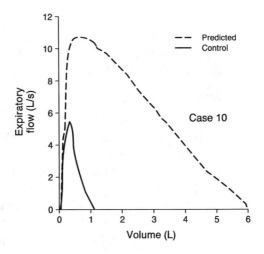

30 y   M   Wt 151 lb (68 kg)   Ht 73 in. (186 cm)

	Normal	Observed	% predicted
Spirometry			
FVC (L)	6.01	1.12*	19
FEV$_1$ (L)	4.89	1.04*	21
FEV$_1$/FVC (%)	81	93	
FEF$_{25-75}$ (L/s)	4.6	2.2*	48
MVV (L/min)	190	81*	43
Volumes			
TLC (L)	7.45	2.09*	28
RV/TLC (%)	19	44*	232
D$_{L_{CO}}$ (mL/min/mm Hg)	35	9*	26

Questions

1. What is your initial impression of the flow-volume curve?
2. Do the data confirm your initial impression?
3. Could obesity or a severe chest wall deformity produce these results?

CASE 10

Answers

1. The initial impression is of severe ventilatory limitation on a restrictive basis because of the marked decrease in the FVC and the steep slope of the flow-volume curve $\left(\text{roughly } 7\dfrac{\text{L/sec}}{\text{L}}\right)$.

2. The extremely low TLC supports a restrictive process as the cause of the limitation. In addition, the markedly reduced $D_{L_{CO}}$ suggests disease of the lung parenchyma. Indeed, this man had severe interstitial fibrosis of unknown cause. He also had cor pulmonale. His oxygen saturation at rest was 95%, and it decreased to 85% with mild stair climbing.

3. Although extreme obesity can reduce the TLC, it probably never does it to this extent. Also, a normal to increased $D_{L_{CO}}$ might be expected in obesity. A severe chest deformity should not be associated with this degree of reduction in the $D_{L_{CO}}$. Furthermore, the steep slope of the flow-volume curve is very unlikely with either extreme obesity or chest wall deformity.

CASE 11

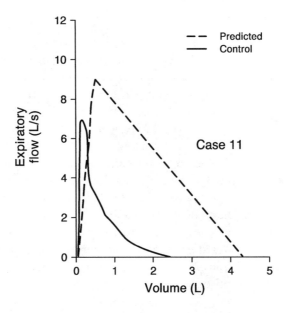

68 y   M   Wt 224 lb (102 kg)   Ht 74 in. (188 cm)

	Normal	Observed	% predicted
Spirometry			
FVC (L)	4.36	2.43*	56
FEV$_1$ (L)	3.05	1.59*	52
FEV$_1$/FVC (%)	70	66	
FEF$_{25-75}$ (L/s)	2.7	0.7*	26
MVV (L/min)	117	87*	75
Volumes			
TLC (L)	7.84	4.95*	63
RV/TLC (%)	44	51	116
D$_{LCO}$ (mL/min/mm Hg)	36	28	78

Questions

1. This 68-year-old man had recently noted becoming quite short of breath when first lying down. Because this then decreased, he was able to sleep at night. He denied any significant dyspnea while walking or climbing stairs. He had been a heavy smoker but quit 15 years ago. What is your initial impression of the flow-volume curve?
2. Do the test results agree with your initial assessment?
3. Are there any other tests you might order?

CASE 11

Answers

1. Certainly the flow-volume curve suggests a moderately severe ventilatory limitation that, on the basis of the contour of the curve, appears to be obstructive in nature.

2. The test results do not totally support the stated diagnosis. There is some airflow obstruction, indicated best by the reduced FEF_{25-75}. However, the reduction in the TLC is not consistent with pure obstruction. The patient's BMI of 28.9 kg/m^2 is not sufficient to explain the restrictive component as being due to obesity.

3. The history suggested to the clinician that the patient might have bilateral diaphragmatic paralysis. He ordered fluoroscopy, which showed paralyzed diaphragms. He also ordered a supine flow-volume curve. Note the marked reduction of the second flow-volume curve obtained in the supine posture.

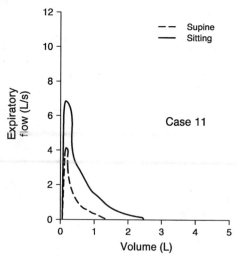

The physician also ordered maximal respiratory pressure measurements:

PEmax was 215 cm H_2O (normal, 200)
PImax was −36 cm H_2O (normal, 103)

These data are consistent with almost complete paralysis of the diaphragm. In summary, this was a limitation due to a mixed restrictive-obstructive process. The restrictive process dominated and was due to idiopathic diaphragmatic paralysis.

CASE 12

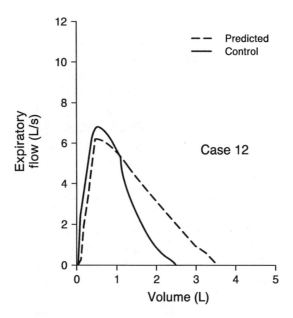

49 y   F   Wt 158 lb (72 kg)   Ht 66 in. (168 cm)

	Normal	Observed	% predicted
Spirometry			
FVC (L)	3.55	2.43	68
FEV$_1$ (L)	2.89	2.20	76
FEV$_1$/FVC (%)	81	91	
FEF$_{25-75}$ (L/s)	2.7	3.3	123
MVV (L/min)	106	92	87
Volumes			
TLC (L)	5.31	4.39	83
RV/TLC (%)	33	36	109
D$_{LCO}$ (mL/min/mm Hg)	23	14*	61

Comments and Questions

The patient complained of dyspnea climbing one flight of stairs. She had never smoked. She had some joint stiffness and pain.

1. What does the flow-volume curve suggest?
2. Considering the test results, what is your final interpretation? (Note that during the past 3 years the TLC, FVC, and D$_{LCO}$ have gradually declined.)

CASE 12

Answers

1. The lost area under the normal curve suggests mild ventilatory limitation. The rather steep slope of the flow-volume curve suggests either a restrictive process or a nonspecific process, depending on the TLC.
2. The mild reduction in the TLC does not quite qualify for a restrictive dysfunction, but it should raise your suspicion. The best interpretation is that of a mild nonspecific ventilatory limitation associated with a reduced diffusing capacity.

The patient has scleroderma with minimal interstitial fibrosis shown by radiography, which explains the reduced $D_{L_{CO}}$ and probably the steep slope of the flow-volume curve. The fibrosis and the chest skin changes of scleroderma are reducing the TLC.

CASE 13

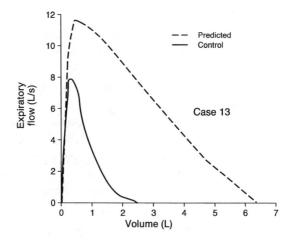

39 y   M   Wt 170 lb (77 kg)   Arm span 79 in. (200 cm)

	Normal	*Observed*	*% predicted*
Spirometry			
FVC (L)	6.32	2.37*	38
FEV$_1$ (L)	5	1.94*	39
FEV$_1$/FVC (%)	79	82	
FEF$_{25-75}$ (L/s)	4.4	1.7*	38
MVV (L/min)	186	121*	65
Volumes			
TLC (L)	7.94	3.62*	46
RV/TLC (%)	20	33	165
D$_{L_{CO}}$ (mL/min/mm Hg)	39	19*	50

Questions

1. How do you classify the flow-volume curve?
2. What is your interpretation after reviewing the test results?
3. What is the diagnosis?

CASE 13

Answers

1. The flow-volume curve can be described as showing severe ventilatory limitation, and the slope of the curve suggests a restrictive component.
2. The reduced TLC confirms the presence of a restrictive defect. In addition, the reduced $D_{L_{CO}}$ suggests a parenchymal abnormality. Therefore, this is a severe ventilatory limitation on the basis of a restrictive process with an impaired diffusing capacity suggesting a parenchymal abnormality.
3. Note that the patient's arm span was used to predict his normal values. The patient has severe idiopathic scoliosis with areas of compressed lung. Use of the measured height would have underestimated the severity of his problem, as seen below.

The flow-volume curve below shows the patient's curve plotted against the predicted curve for his actual height of 167.6 cm. Now the FVC is 54% of predicted versus 38%, and the FEV_1 shows a similar difference.

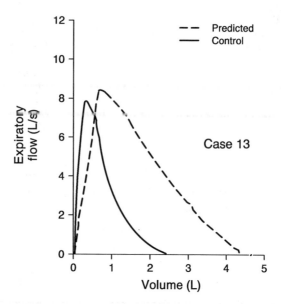

This is a complex case. The main point is that the technicians must measure the arm span and use it to predict the normal values in all subjects with spinal deformities.

CASE 14

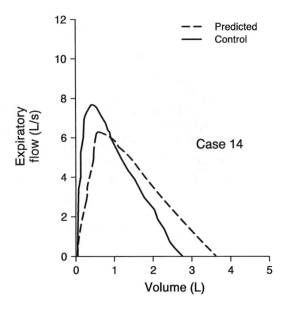

22 y F Wt 117 lb (53 kg) Ht 60 in. (152 cm)

	Normal	Observed	% predicted	Post-dilator
Spirometry				
FVC (L)	3.63	2.83*	78	2.65
FEV$_1$ (L)	3.21	2.58*	81	2.49
FEV$_1$/FVC (%)	88	92		
FEF$_{25-75}$ (L/s)	3.7	3.8	103	
MVV (L/min)	118	88	75	
Volumes				
TLC (L)	4.45	3.6	81	
RV/TLC (%)	18	22	122	
D$_{LCO}$ (mL/min/mm Hg)	24	23	93	

Comments and Questions

This 22-year-old woman was seen for a lump in her throat that interfered with swallowing and for anxiety. She noted in passing that
sometimes she became short of breath, but she denied wheezing.
Results of physical examination were negative.

1. How would you interpret the flow-volume curve and test
   data?
2. Is there any other procedure you would order?

CASE 14

Answers

1. On the basis of the area loss at lower volumes, the low-normal TLC, the proportional reduction in FVC and FEV_1 resulting in a normal ratio, the lack of a dilator response, and the normal DL_{CO}, this test fits the "nonspecific ventilatory limitation" category. Airway resistance was measured and was normal.

2. Because the results of cardiac examination were normal and the cause of her dyspnea was unknown, a methacholine challenge test was ordered. The curve after five breaths of methacholine is shown below. There was a 35% decrease in the FEV_1 associated with chest tightness and dyspnea similar to what the patient had been experiencing.

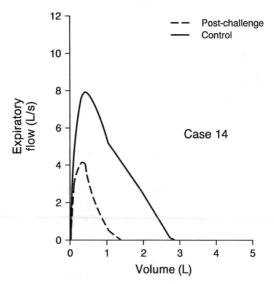

An interesting feature is the parallel shift in the post-methacholine curve resulting in an FEV_1/FVC ratio that was 90% despite the severe bronchoconstriction. Also, the measurement of airway resistance during the initial part of the study failed to detect any abnormality. The slightly increased slope of the control curve and the low-normal TLC might raise the question of mild pulmonary fibrosis but, of course, the normal DL_{CO} argues against this. In fact, this is an example of occult asthma characterized mainly by a decrease in the FVC and some increase in the slope of the flow-volume curve.

CASE 15

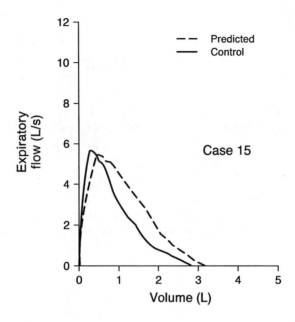

64 y   F   Wt 377 lb (171 kg)   Ht 65 in. (165 cm)

	Normal	*Observed*	*% predicted*	*Post-dilator*
Spirometry				
FVC (L)	3.13	2.89	92	2.81
FEV$_1$ (L)	2.48	2.15	87	2.1
FEV$_1$/FVC (%)	80	74		
FEF$_{25-75}$ (L/s)	2.2	1.6	73	
MVV (L/min)	94	90	96	
DL$_{CO}$ (mL/min/mm Hg)	21	25	119	

Question

1.   How would you interpret this test?

CASE 15

Answer

1. The loss of area suggests mild ventilatory limitation despite the normal data. The interpretation would be possible mild ventilatory limitation on a nonspecific basis. The contour of the flow-volume curve suggests mild airway obstruction. Measurement of TLC would be needed to determine whether a restrictive component is present. The patient's excessive weight for her height may be playing a role in the mild limitation.

This case illustrates that even in an elderly nonsmoker, morbid obesity (the BMI is 62.8 kg/m^2) may have only a mild effect on pulmonary function. Of course, this is not always the case.

CASE 16

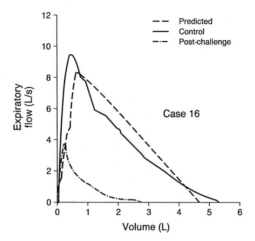

17 y   M   Wt 170 lb (77 kg)   Ht 69 in. (175 cm)

	Normal	Observed	% predicted	Post-challenge	% change
Spirometry					
FVC (L)	4.67	5.37	115	2.72	−49
FEV$_1$ (L)	4.02	3.88	96	1.45	−63
FEV$_1$/FVC (%)	86	72*		53	
FEF$_{25-75}$ (L/s)	4.5	2.8	63	0.6	
MVV (L/min)	161	144	89		
Volumes					
TLC (L)	6.06	6.68	110		
RV/TLC (%)	19	20	105		
D$_{L_{CO}}$ (mL/min/ mm Hg)	32	30	95		

Comments

This young man has had asthma and hay fever since age 6 years. He also has exercise-induced asthma and is allergic to certain seafood.

He is presented here to show how extreme the response can be to one breath of methacholine (5 mg/mL). The control curve suggests borderline ventilatory limitation on an obstructive basis, the slope of the flow-volume curve being decreased and the FEV$_1$/FVC ratio slightly reduced. The other test results are normal, and on the basis of these results one would not expect the 63% decrease in the FEV$_1$, which was associated with wheezing and significant dyspnea.

CASE 17

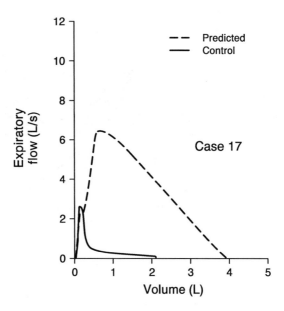

29 y   F   Wt 110 lb (50 kg)   Ht 65 in. (165 cm)

	Normal	Observed	% predicted	Post-dilator
Spirometry				
FVC (L)	3.93	2.39*	61	2.86
FEV$_1$ (L)	3.34	0.62*	19	0.67
FEV$_1$/FVC (%)	85	26*		
FEF$_{25-75}$ (L/s)	3.4	0.2*	6	0.2
MVV (L/min)	119	28*	23	
Volumes				
TLC (L)	5.18	6.63	128	
RV/TLC (%)	24	59*	246	
D$_{L_{CO}}$ (mL/min/mm Hg)	25	7*	28	

Questions

1. How would you grade the limitation based on the flow-volume curve?
2. Do the spirometry results support your impression? (The post-dilator curve is not shown because it could not be distinguished from the control curve.)
3. Are the volumes and $D_{L_{CO}}$ also consistent?
4. What is unusual about this case?

CASE 17

Answers

1. The flow-volume curve shows severe ventilatory limitation due to an obstructive process. The shape of the curve is characteristic of obstruction.
2. Spirometry results are consistent with severe obstruction.
3. The high normal TLC and reduced DL_{CO} are consistent. The low DL_{CO} suggests a parenchymal abnormality such as emphysema.
4. The patient was a nonsmoker with no history of asthma. This degree of obstruction in such a young person is rare. One possibility would be α_1-antitrypsin deficiency, but results of blood tests were normal. On open-lung biopsy, the patient was found to have lymphangioleiomyomatosis. This is a rare disease in which there is proliferation of atypical smooth muscle throughout the peribronchial, perivascular, and perilymphatic regions of the lung. Pulmonary infiltrates were prominent on chest radiography (these do not occur in α_1-antitrypsin deficiency) and contribute to the reduction in the DL_{CO}.

CASE 18

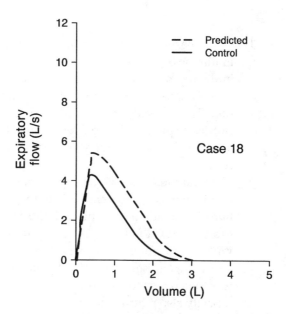

73 y   F   Wt 150 lb (68 kg)   Ht 64 in. (162 cm)

	Normal	*Observed*	*% predicted*
Spirometry			
FVC (L)	3.19	2.72	85
FEV$_1$ (L)	2.33	1.83	79
FEV$_1$/FVC (%)	79	67	
FEF$_{25-75}$ (L/s)	1.9	1.7	89
MVV (L/min)	88	81	92
D$_{L_{CO}}$ (mL/min/mm Hg)	18	9.4*	52

Comments and Questions

This 73-year-old woman complained of cough for 2 months. The cough had begun after a flu-like illness. She was a nonsmoker. She denied wheezing and dyspnea. On examination, her lungs were clear. She had a grade 4/6 harsh precordial systolic murmur.

1. How would you interpret this test? (She did not show any response to inhaled bronchodilator.)
2. What might be the cause of her problem?

CASE 18

Answers

1. On the basis of the area comparison, there is mild ventilatory limitation of a nonspecific nature, the FEV_1/FVC ratio being in the normal range. However, the terminal portion of the flow-volume curve suggests the presence of mild obstruction. The markedly reduced diffusing capacity suggests a restrictive process due to a lung parenchymal abnormality, but because there is not a measure of TLC, this cannot be confirmed.

2. The loud murmur was the important clue. Her chest radiograph showed an interstitial pattern (easily confused with fibrosis), small bilateral pleural effusions, and an enlarged heart. Results of electrocardiography were also abnormal. With therapy for the congestive heart failure, her cough disappeared, and she lost 12 lb. The flow-volume curve below was then obtained. It was totally normal, and the diffusing capacity also returned to normal.

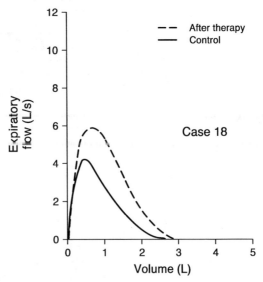

Congestive heart failure can present with cough as the only significant complaint. The pulmonary function test can mimic a restrictive process due to congested lymphatics and perivascular and peribronchial edema. Comparison of the flow-volume curves indicates that initially mild obstruction was present. Sometimes this can be quite marked and lead to "cardiac asthma."

CASE 19

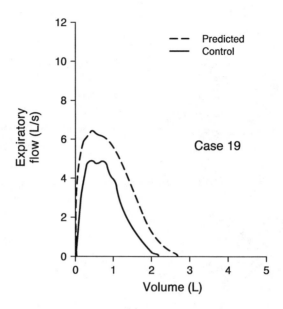

40 y   F   Wt 213 lb (97 kg)   Ht 62 in. (157 cm)

	Normal	Observed	% predicted
Spirometry			
FVC (L)	3.32	2.14*	64
FEV$_1$ (L)	2.59	1.94*	75
FEV$_1$/FVC (%)	77	90	
FEF$_{25-75}$ (L/s)	3.07	2.72	89
MVV (L/min)	107	79	74
Volumes			
TLC (L)	4.65	4.02	86
RV/TLC (%)	32	35	109

Comments and Questions

The patient gave a 4-year history of episodes of shortness of breath. Typically, she awoke in the morning with dyspnea and no wheezing, but some nocturnal cough. Attacks would subside in 1 to 2 days, and she knew of nothing that precipitated them. She was a nonsmoker. Results of physical examination were unremarkable. The lungs were clear, and the heart was normal.

1. What is your interpretation of this test?
2. What do you think the problem is?
3. Are there any other procedures you would order?

CASE 19

Answers

1. The proportionate reduction in the FVC and FEV_1 with a normal FEV_1/FVC ratio suggests a restrictive process. However, the normal TLC essentially rules out restriction. Thus, "mild ventilatory limitation on a nonspecific basis" is the remaining possibility.
2. As shown previously, a normal FEV_1/FVC ratio does not rule out obstruction. Because of the nocturnal nature of the patient's symptoms, you may have suspected asthma.
3. If you ordered a bronchodilator, you were correct. As can be seen from the flow-volume curves below, the post-dilator curve is normal. The FEV_1 increased by 25%.

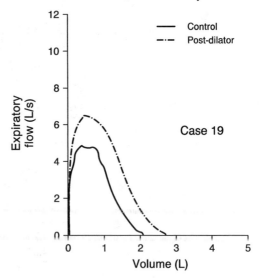

This case reinforces several points:

Not all asthma wheezes.

Asthma is often a nocturnal disorder.

The patient's excess weight for her height (BMI is 39 kg/m^2) may have tended to make the TLC a bit low.

This is another example of the FEV_1/FVC ratio not being an infallible test of obstruction.

The two flow-volume curves really show a parallel shift, as is often seen in mild asthma. In these instances, the FEV_1/FVC ratio does not decrease until obstruction increases to a significant degree.

CASE 20

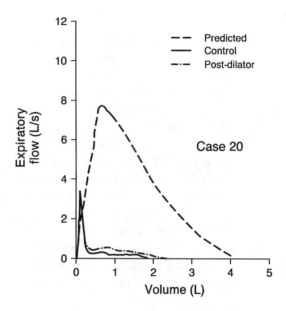

69 y   M   Wt 143 lb (65 kg)   Ht 68 in. (173 cm)

	Normal	Observed	% predicted	Post-dilator
Spirometry				
FVC (L)	4.11	1.73*	42	2.30*
FEV$_1$ (L)	3.18	0.48*	15	0.63*
FEV$_1$/FVC (%)	77	28*		
FEF$_{25-75}$ (L/s)	2.8	0.2*	8	0.3*
MVV (L/min)	124	24*	19	
Volumes				
TLC (L)	6.39	7.62	119	
RV/TLC (%)	36	71*	197	
D$_{L_{CO}}$ (mL/min/mm Hg)	25	12*	47	

Questions

1. How would you interpret this test?
2. What would you predict the pre-dilator MVV would be?

CASE 20

Answers

1. This is a classic case of severe obstructive disease. There is a small response to bronchodilator. The reduced $D_{L_{CO}}$ suggests an element of anatomic emphysema. The plateau in the flow-volume curve is typical of severe chronic obstructive pulmonary disease and should not be mistaken for a variable intrathoracic airway lesion.

2. The pre-dilator MVV would be predicted to be 40×0.48 (FEV_1) = 19 L/min. The measured value was 24 L/min. This difference does not mean that the FEV_1 was in error but merely points out the limitation of the prediction equation and the variability in the relationship between the MVV and FEV_1. Of interest, during an exercise study done on the same day, the patient achieved a minute ventilation of 36 L/min. Thus, predicting maximal ventilation during exercise from the FEV_1 or MVV may also not be exact.

CASE 21

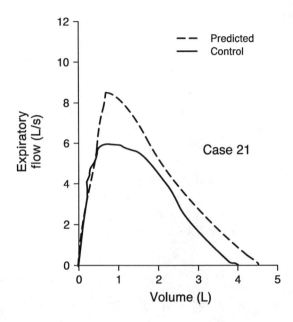

50 y   M   Wt 161 lb (73 kg)   Ht 68 in. (173 cm)

Spirometry	Normal	Observed	% predicted
FVC (L)	4.61	4.02	87
FEV$_1$ (L)	3.69	3.23	88
FEV$_1$/FVC (%)	80	80	
FEF$_{25-75}$ (L/s)	3.4	3.0	88
MVV (L/min)	150	46*	31

Comments and Questions

This patient complained of dyspnea on climbing stairs. He was a nonsmoker. Results of cardiac examination were negative. Auscultation revealed some decrease in breath sounds. Nineteen years previously he had had bulbar poliomyelitis, from which he recovered completely. No improvement was seen after he was given a bronchodilator.

1. What is your interpretation?
2. Is there any other procedure you would order?

CASE 21

Answers

1. There is a slight loss of area, suggesting a mild nonspecific limitation. The contour of the flow-volume curve is normal. However, there is an isolated, significant reduction in the MVV. This might reflect a major airway lesion, a neuromuscular problem, or submaximal patient effort.
2. Because the technician thought the patient made a maximal effort on the MVV, you should order an inspiratory flow-volume curve. This was obtained (shown below) and indicated that the patient had a variable extrathoracic major airway lesion. This was due to total paralysis of the right vocal cord and partial paralysis of the left, which resulted in an orifice-like constriction during inspiration.

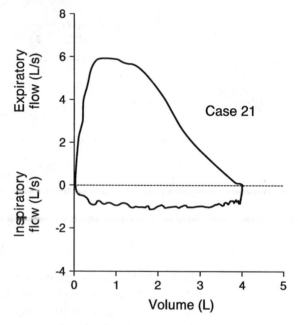

The tip-off to the diagnosis was the unexplained reduction in the MVV with what seemed to be a good effort. On the basis of the FEV_1, you would expect the MVV to be about 129 L/min (3.23 × 40). Thus, this was a striking reduction. However, if the inspiratory flow-volume loop was normal, you would then order maximal respiratory pressure measurements.

CASE 22

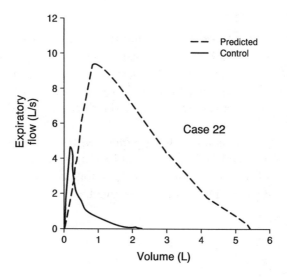

68 y   M   Wt 217 lb (99 kg)   Ht 74 in. (188 cm)

	Normal	Observed	% predicted	Post-dilator
Spirometry				
FVC (L)	5.46	2.33*	43	2.2
FEV$_1$ (L)	4.10	1.17*	28	1.19
FEV$_1$/FVC (%)	75	50*		
FEF$_{25-75}$ (L/s)	3.3	0.4*	12	0.4
MVV (L/min)	145	50*	34	
Volumes				
TLC (L)	7.69	4.74*	62	
RV/TLC (%)	29	46*	159	
D$_{LCO}$ (mL/min/mm Hg)	28	17*	60	

Question

1. How would you interpret the results?

CASE 22

Answer

1. There is severe ventilatory limitation on a mixed obstructive and restrictive basis. The restriction is reflected in the reduced TLC. The obstruction is reflected in the decreased expiratory flows and increased curvature of the flow-volume curve. There is a mild reduction of the diffusing capacity.

This is an unusual pattern with severe obstruction and yet a reduced TLC. The patient had undergone a left pneumonectomy 10 years previously for squamous cell lung cancer. Considering this, the DL_{CO} is well preserved.

CASE 23

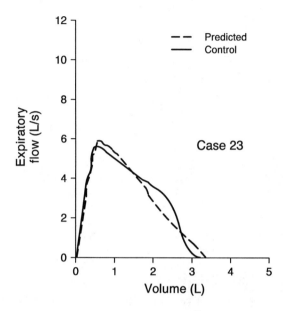

45 y   F   Wt 131 lb (60 kg)   Ht 62 in. (157 cm)

Spirometry	Normal	Observed	% predicted	Post-dilator
FVC (L)	3.44	3.96	115	4.0
FEV$_1$ (L)	2.84	2.98	105	
FEV$_1$/FVC (%)	82	75		
FEF$_{25-75}$ (L/s)	2.7	3.51	130	
MVV (L/min)	106	122	115	

Comments and Questions

The patient is a 45-year-old woman who for the past 1 to 2 years had noted dyspnea when hurrying on the level or when climbing stairs. She had noted slight arm weakness.

1. What is your interpretation of this test?
2. Is there any other test you would order?

CASE 23

Answers

1. The study results are normal. The shape of the flow-volume curve suggests that the patient was a nonsmoker, which, indeed, she was.
2. Did you order maximal respiratory pressure measurements? Unexplained dyspnea and slight muscle weakness should alert you to the possibility of an early neuromuscular disorder.

	Normal	Observed	% of normal
PImax (cm H_2O)	−70	−26*	37
PEmax (cm H_2O)	135	90*	67

The maximal inspiratory pressure was more reduced than the expiratory pressure. Eventually, amyotrophic lateral sclerosis was diagnosed. This is an example of dyspnea due to muscle weakness appearing at a time when spirometry results were still normal.

CASE 24

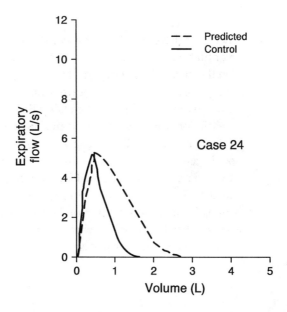

72 y   F   Wt 249 lb (113 kg)   Ht 63 in. (160 cm)

	Normal	Observed	% predicted
Spirometry			
FVC (L)	2.75	1.56*	57
FEV_1 (L)	2.18	1.34*	62
FEV_1/FVC (%)	79	86	
FEF_{25-75} (L/s)	2	1.7	
MVV (L/min)	86	53*	62
Volumes			
TLC (L)	4.88	3.77*	77
RV/TLC (%)	44	51	116
DL_{CO} (mL/min/mm Hg)	20	16	79

Question

1. What is your interpretation of the results in this 72-year-old nonsmoking woman?

CASE 24

Answer

1. Because there is a loss of area, she has mild to moderate ventilatory limitation. The limitation is restrictive in nature on the basis of the reduced TLC. Although the flow-volume curve is a bit steep, the normal $D_{L_{CO}}$ is against a significant parenchymal process causing the restriction. Thus, the restriction is extrapulmonary and most likely due to the patient's obesity, her BMI being 44.1 kg/m^2. This case contrasts with case 15 (page 173), in which even more massive obesity caused no reduction in the FVC and presumably no change in the TLC. On average, obesity with a BMI kg/m^2 more than 35 causes a reduction of 5% to 10% in FVC, but the effect of obesity is highly variable. It may be marked, as in this case, or negligible, as in case 15.

CASE 25

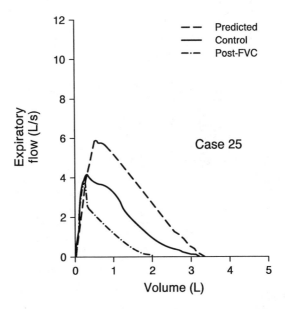

42 y   F   Wt 152 lb (69 kg)   Ht 62 in. (157 cm)

	Normal	Observed	% predicted	Post-FVC
Spirometry				
FVC (L)	3.32	3.34	101	2.11*
FEV$_1$ (L)	2.81	2.16*	77	1.46*
FEV$_1$/FVC (%)	85	65*		
FEF$_{25-75}$ (L/s)	5.9	4.2	71	
MVV (L/min)	106	41*	39	
Volumes				
TLC (L)	4.69	4.26	91	
RV/TLC (%)	1.37	0.92	67	
D$_{L_{CO}}$ (mL/min/mm Hg)	23	18	77	

Comments

The control flow-volume curve and data are consistent with mild to perhaps moderate airway obstruction. After the control FVC maneuver, however, audible wheezing developed and the post-FVC curve was obtained. FEV$_1$ was reduced by 32%. This is an example of FVC-induced bronchoconstriction, which sometimes occurs in patients with hyperreactive airways, such as in asthma. The MVV is reduced because of the induced bronchospasm.

CASE 26

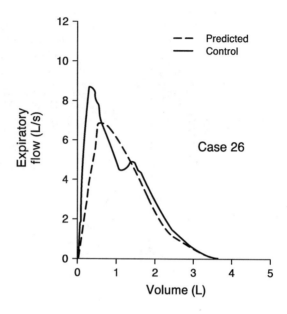

86 y   M   Wt 137 lb (62 kg)   Ht 67 in. (170 cm)

	Normal	*Observed*	*% predicted*	*Post-dilator*
Spirometry				
FVC (L)	3.6	3.85	107	3.95
FEV$_1$ (L)	2.7	2.87	106	2.66
FEV$_1$/FVC (%)	75	75		
FEF$_{25-75}$ (L/s)	2.4	2.2	92	
MVV (L/min)	100	83	83	
Volumes				
TLC (L)	6.24	5.71	92	
RV/TLC (%)	42	31	74	
D$_{LCO}$ (mL/min/mm Hg)	21	4*	20	

Comment and Questions

This is a case of an isolated reduction in the $D_{L_{CO}}$.

1. What might be the cause of this finding?
2. Is there any significance to the contour of the flow-volume curve?

CASE 26

Answers

1. A poor effort or equipment problems could cause this low value. However, the test was repeated on a different unit and was not changed. The patient was not anemic, but severe anemia could contribute to a reduced $D_{L_{CO}}$. The tests showed no evidence of emphysema. The chest radiograph did show an extensive fine interstitial infiltrate thought to represent metastatic cancer. The mildly reduced RV/TLC ratio might reflect an early restrictive process, but essentially the volumes and spirometry results are normal.

2. The notch in the flow-volume curve was not seen on other efforts and is of no significance.

CASE 27

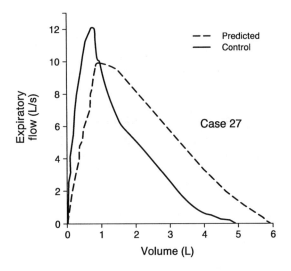

42 y   M   Wt 214 lb (97 kg)   Ht 74 in. (188 cm)

	Normal	Observed	% predicted	Post-dilator
Spirometry				
FVC (L)	5.91	5.15	87	5.10
FEV$_1$ (L)	4.68	3.82*	82	3.87
FEV$_1$/FVC (%)	79	74		
FEF$_{25-75}$ (L/s)	4.1	2.8	67	
MVV (L/min)	177	174	99	
Volumes				
TLC (L)	7.60	7.75	102	
RV/TLC (%)	22	30*		
D$_{Lco}$ (mL/min/mm Hg)	34	56	163	

Questions

1. How would you interpret this study? (The patient is a moderate smoker.)
2. What is particularly unusual, and what might be the cause?

CASE 27

Answers

1. The flow-volume curve shows mild ventilatory limitation, and the contour suggests airway obstruction. The reduced FEV_1 is consistent with this impression.

2. The unusual feature is the remarkable increase in the D_{LCO}. Such an increase can occur in asthma, obesity, and polycythemia. The patient had an atrial septal defect with a significant left-to-right shunt. This produced an increased pulmonary capillary blood volume and, hence, the high D_{LCO}.

CASE 28

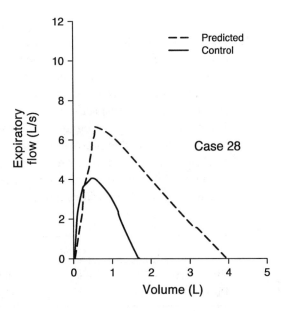

31 y   F   Wt 105 lb (48 kg)   Ht 65 in. (165 cm)

	Normal	Observed	% predicted	Post-dilator
Spirometry				
FVC (L)	3.94	1.73*	44	1.67
FEV$_1$ (L)	3.32	1.67*	50	1.62
FEV$_1$/FVC (%)	84	96		
FEF$_{25-75}$ (L/s)	3.3	3.1	93	
MVV (L/min)	119	58*	49	
Volumes				
TLC (L)	5.26	5.43	103	
RV/TLC (%)	25	68*		
D$_{L_{CO}}$ (mL/min/mm Hg)	25	29	114	

Questions

1. How would you interpret this test?
2. Do the flow-volume curve and test data suggest the need for other tests?

CASE 28

Answers

1. There is significant ventilatory limitation (that is, loss of area under the flow-volume curve). The curve is steep, but the normal TLC and diffusing capacity rule out a pulmonary parenchymal restrictive process. At this point, this case can be classified as a nonspecific abnormality.
2. There are no findings to suggest a major airway lesion. However, another possible cause of such a pattern is a neuromuscular problem. If you thought maximal respiratory pressures should be determined to assess respiratory muscle strength, you were correct. The values follow:

	Normal	Patient	% normal
PImax (cm H_2O)	−88	−64*	30
PEmax (cm H_2O)	154	113*	23

The patient has severe amyotrophic lateral sclerosis. The muscle weakness led to the decreased FVC and FEV_1 and the increased RV/TLC ratio. Surprisingly, a normal TLC was maintained. Compare this case to case 23 (page 189), a less severe case of muscle weakness.

CASE 29

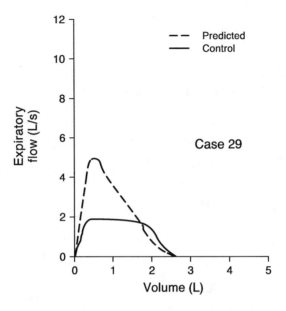

64 y   F   Wt 142 lb (64 kg)   Ht 60 in. (152 cm)

Spirometry	Normal	Observed	% predicted	Post-dilator
FVC (L)	2.60	2.76	106	2.70
FEV$_1$ (L)	2.13	1.84	86	1.85
FEV$_1$/FVC (%)	82	67	82	69
FEF$_{25-75}$ (L/s)	2.2	2	91	
MVV (L/min)	87	27*	31	

Comment and Question

This nonsmoker complained of the gradual onset over 5 years of dyspnea on exertion, often associated with noisy breathing.

1. What is your preliminary diagnosis, and how would you proceed?

CASE 29

Answer

1. The history, shape of the flow-volume curve, and isolated
   reduction in MVV should make you think "major airway
   lesion." Then, a flow-volume loop would be ordered, which
   is shown in the figure below.

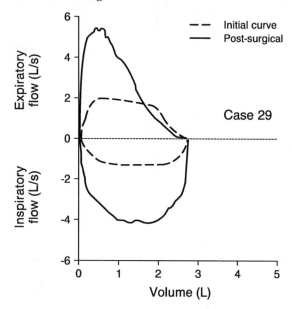

The patient had an idiopathic subglottic stenosis leading to the
pattern of a fixed major airway lesion. The stricture was removed,
and the postoperative flow-volume loop was normal.

CASE 30

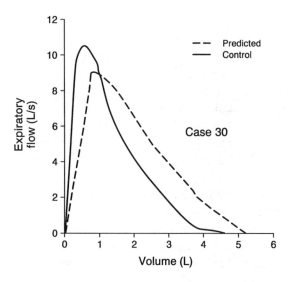

31 y   M   Wt 226 lb (103 kg)   Ht 72 in. (182 cm)

	Normal	*Observed*	*% predicted*
Spirometry			
FVC (L)	5.23	4.43	85
FEV$_1$ (L)	4.12	3.48	84
FEV$_1$/FVC (%)	79	78	
FEF$_{25-75}$ (L/s)	3.6	2.6	73
MVV (L/min)	158	137	87
Volumes			
TLC (L)	7.11	7.38	104
RV/TLC (%)	27	36*	
DL$_{CO}$ (mL/min/mm Hg)	33	26	79
O$_2$ saturation (%)			
Rest	96	90*	
Exercise	96	85*	

Questions

1. Is there anything in the data to explain the subject's desaturation?
2. Can you rule out some possible causes?

CASE 30

Answers

1. Nothing in the data indicates the cause of the subject's desaturation. The mild increase in the RV/TLC ratio is not helpful.
2. The flow-volume curve shows borderline ventilatory limitation, but nothing indicates the cause of the problem. The TLC and $D_{L_{CO}}$ effectively rule out lung parenchymal disease. The patient is mildly overweight (BMI is 31.1 kg/m^2), but the weight is not severe enough to cause this problem.

The patient had advanced liver disease with small intrathoracic right-to-left shunts causing the desaturation. The patient exhibited orthodeoxia; namely, the saturation decreased when he went from the recumbent to the standing position. He underwent liver transplantation, which was successful, and the desaturation was abolished.

CASE 31

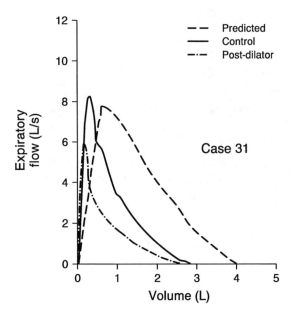

46 y   M   Wt 246 lb (112 kg)   Ht 65 in. (165 cm)

	Normal	Observed	% predicted	Post-dilator
Spirometry				
FVC (L)	4	3.07*	77	2.76
FEV$_1$ (L)	3.27	2.23*	68	1.68
FEV$_1$/FVC (%)	82	73		61
FEF$_{25-75}$ (L/s)	3.3	1.5	46	
MVV (L/min)	145	90*	62	
Volumes				
TLC (L)	5.81	5.5	95	
RV/TLC (%)	31	41*		
D$_{LCO}$ (mL/min/mm Hg)	29	33	112	

Question

1. How would you interpret the test results?

CASE 31

Answer

1. The first thing you should note is that the post-dilator flow-volume curve is lower than the control curve. This is a paradoxical response to isoproterenol (Isuprel), and a fairly rare occurrence. When the patient was tested later with albuterol, there was not such a decrease in flows and some improvement was seen in the curve. In addition, the control curve shows mild ventilatory limitation. The "scooping" of the flow-volume curve and the increased RV/TLC ratio suggest an obstructive process. The patient is obese (BMI is 41.1 kg/m^2). This may contribute to the reduction in FVC and FEV$_1$.

CASE 32

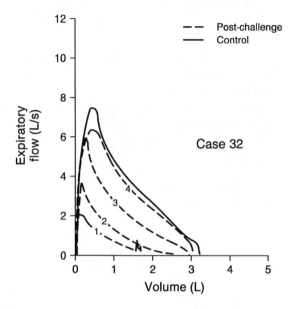

14 y   F   Wt 110 lb (50 kg)   Ht 64 in. (162 cm)

	Normal	Observed	% predicted
Spirometry			
FVC (L)	3.28	3.28	100
FEV$_1$ (L)	2.9	2.93	101
FEV$_1$/FVC (%)	88	89	
FEF$_{25-75}$ (L/s)	3.5	3.1	88
MVV (L/min)	116	117	101
Volumes			
TLC (L)	4.5	4.3	96
RV/TLC (%)	19	21	
D$_{LCO}$ (mL/min/mm Hg)	23	23	100

Comments

The baseline data are all normal. Because of the patient's history of intermittent wheezing and shortness of breath, a methacholine challenge test was performed. The patient inhaled five breaths of methacholine and her flows promptly decreased (curve 1), and the FEV$_1$ decreased 62%. As repeated FVCs were obtained, the bronchospasm progressively decreased, and eventually the FEV$_1$ was reduced by only 14%, which is usually considered a negative test result. However, in this situation, it seems clear that the patient has hyperreactive airways. In this case, the mere effort of inhaling to TLC decreased the degree of bronchoconstriction, a relatively unusual event.

Also note the terminal portion of the control flow-volume curve. At approximately 3.2 L exhaled volume, the flow decreases precipitously to zero. As shown in Fig. 2-6E (page 16), such a curve can be a normal variant, as in this case. With bronchoconstriction, this feature is lost, but it is seen again as the bronchoconstriction subsides (see determinants of RV, page 30 and the second Pearl, page 39).

CASE 33

36 y   F   Wt 211 lb (95.5 kg)   Ht 63 in. (160 cm)

	Normal	Observed	% predicted
Spirometry			
FVC (L)	3.57	1.90*	53
FEV$_1$ (L)	3.02	0.72*	24
FEV$_1$/FVC (%)	85	38*	
FEF$_{25-75}$ (L/s)	3.1	0.8*	26
MVV (L/min)	100	58*	58
Volumes			
TLC (L)	5.20	4.91	94
RV/TLC (%)	30	61*	
DL$_{CO}$ (mL/min/mm Hg)	24	11*	46

Comments and Questions

This 36-year-old woman had noted progressive shortness of breath during the past 6 years. She was a nonsmoker and had no history of asthma or a family history of lung disease. The chest radiograph revealed diffuse interstitial infiltrates. There was no response to bronchodilator.

1. What is your impression based on the above data?
2. Are there aspects of the data that are unusual?
3. Are there additional tests that might be informative?

CASE 33

Answers

1. This is a puzzling case. There is obstruction reflected in the flow-volume curve contour and the very low FEV_1, FEF_{25-75}, and FEV_1/FVC and the increased RV/TLC. The TLC is not increased, which is unusual with this degree of obstruction. The low D_{LCO} and the chest radiograph suggest a possible restrictive component.
2. Lung mechanics testing was performed. Resistance was increased threefold, whereas CL_{stat} was reduced to 56% of predicted and CL_{dyn} to 30% predicted. The graphic data emphasize the lack of hyperinflation, the low maximal expiratory flows, and the relatively normal lung recoil curve. The resulting MFSR curve is consistent with extensive airway disease.

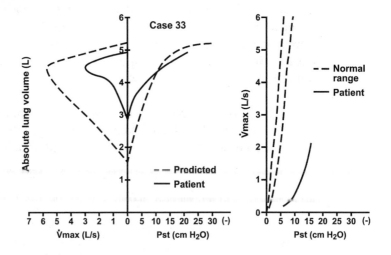

3. A lung biopsy helped with the diagnosis of lymphangioleiomyomatosis. In this case, despite the severe obstruction, there was no increase in either the TLC or CL_{stat}, a very unusual situation, which often occurs in this disease (see page 113, and case 17, page 176).

CASE 34

62 y   F   Wt 90 lb (40 kg)   Ht 63 in. (160 cm)

	Normal	Observed	% predicted	Post-dilator
Spirometry				
FVC (L)	2.6	1.95*	75	1.95
FEV$_1$ (L)	1.9	0.35*	18	0.35
FEV$_1$/FVC (%)	74	18*		
FEF$_{25-75}$ (L/s)	2.9	0.3*	10	
MVV (L/min)	62	16*	25	
Volumes				
TLC (L)	4.6	5.5	120	
RV/TLC (%)	43	66*	153	
D$_{Lco}$ (mL/min/mm Hg)	22	8*	36	

Comments and Questions

This 62-year-old woman complained of weight loss, rectal bleeding, nervousness, and some shortness of breath on exertion. She noted dyspnea after having the Hong Kong flu. She had never smoked and had no family history of respiratory disease. The chest radiograph revealed cystic changes at both bases. The TLC measured with the nitrogen washout technique was 1 liter less than that with the plethysmographic TLC reported here.

1. How would you describe these data?
2. Are there any additional tests you would order?

CASE 34

Answers

1. The test results are consistent with severe airway obstruction with hyperinflation, yet dyspnea was not a major complaint. The chest radiograph and the low diffusing capacity suggest the presence of emphysema.

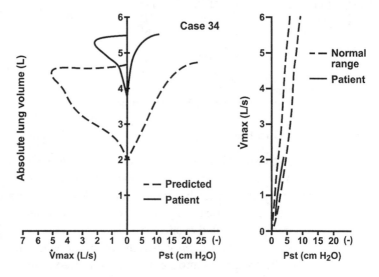

2. A test for α_1-antitrypsin deficiency revealed she was homozygous for the Z gene. Special mechanics studies were ordered. Note the severe loss of lung recoil and hyperinflation. The MFSR curve lies in the normal range, consistent with the condition being pure emphysema. CL_{stat} was increased (0.389 L/cm H_2O), whereas CL_{dyn} was low (0.132 L/cm H_2O) (see section 7B, page 79). Resistance was increased at 6.2 cm H_2O/L/s.

CASE 35

56 y   M   Wt 162 lb (73.6 kg)   Ht 66 in. (168 cm)

	Normal	Observed	% predicted	Post-dilator
Spirometry				
FVC (L)	3.3	4.67	141	4.67
FEV$_1$ (L)	2.4	1.72*	72	2.02
FEV$_1$/FVC (%)	73	37*		
FEF$_{25-75}$ (L/s)	3.4	0.7*	21	
MVV (L/min)	103	79*	79	
Volumes				
TLC (L)	5.7	8.1*	142	
RV/TLC (%)	42	42	101	
D$_{L_{CO}}$ (mL/min/mm Hg)	27	26	96	

Comments and Questions

This 56-year-old man had a 4-year history of progressive dyspnea on exertion. He reported a productive morning cough and occasional wheezing. He had a 30 pack-year history of cigarette smoking. Coarse inspiratory and expiratory wheezes and rhonchi were heard. The chest radiograph was normal. Arterial blood gas tests at rest showed an O_2 saturation of 93%, Pao$_2$ 64 mm Hg, Paco$_2$ 33 mm Hg, and pH 7.52.

1. How would you classify these data?
2. Are there any concerns you have about these data?
3. Are there other data you would like to have?

CASE 35

Answers

1. There is a mild-to-moderate degree of airway obstruction with a good FEV_1 response (17%) to bronchodilator. The normal DL_{CO} is not compatible with an extensive degree of emphysema.
2. Note that the patient was hyperventilating (low $Paco_2$ and increased pH) when the arterial sample was drawn.
3. To rule out emphysema, a mechanics study was done (see below). Note that despite the hyperinflation, the lung recoil is normal and the MFSR curve is to the right of the normal range, indicating that airway disease (chronic bronchitis) was the cause of the low expiratory flows. Rpulm was high (5.0 cm $H_2O/L/s$), CL_{stat} was normal (0.250 L/cm H_2O), and CL_{dyn} was low (0.133 L/cm H_2O).

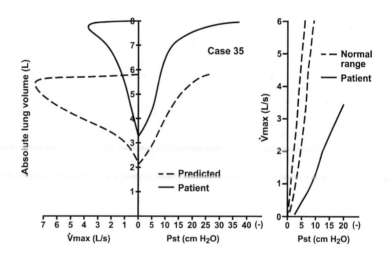

CASE 36

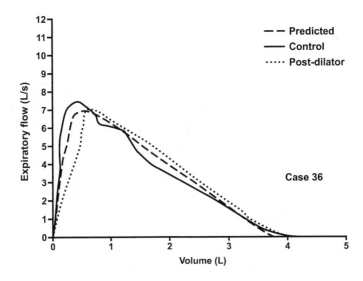

18 y   F   Wt 126 lb (57 kg)   Ht 64 in. (162 cm)

	Normal	Observed	% predicted	Post-dilator
Spirometry				
FVC (L)	3.59	4.06	113	4.06
FEV$_1$ (L)	3.26	3.40	104	3.51
FEV$_1$/FVC (%)	90.8	80	93	
FEF$_{25-75}$ (L/s)	4	3.6	88	
MVV (L/min)	131	127	97	
Volumes				
TLC (L)	4.57	4.94	108	
RV/TLC (%)	19.4	17		
D$_{L_{CO}}$ (mL/min/mm Hg)	24	30	123	

Questions

1. What is your interpretation?
2. The patient had a history of colds with some wheezing. Is there anything else that should be done?

CASE 36

Answers

1. The test is normal. Note the high-normal $D_{L_{CO}}$ and the flattening of the terminal portion of the control flow-volume curve. These may be subtle signs of underlying asthma.

2. Because of the history, you probably ordered a methacholine challenge test. The test was strongly positive after one breath of 25 mg/mL methacholine.

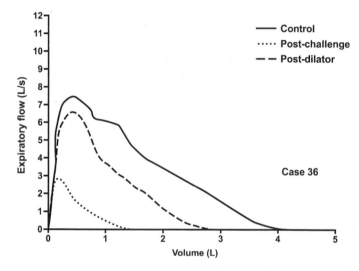

This case illustrates the importance of considering the reactivity of the airways at the time of testing. When the first test was done, the airways were fully dilated and there was no response to bronchodilator. Hence, methacholine was needed to confirm the diagnosis. In some situations, the airways may be constricted such that methacholine will have no effect but a dilator will. In this case, the control FEV_1/FVC ratio was 80%, during the 67% reduction in FEV_1 the ratio was 76%, and it was 81% on the post-dilator curve. This shows that the ratio does not always detect airway obstruction.

CASE 37

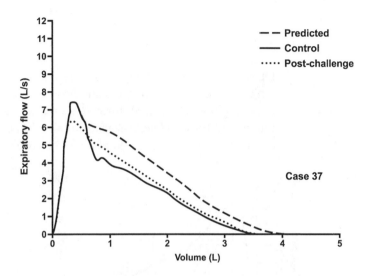

45 y   F   Wt 265 lb (119 kg)   Ht 65.8 in. (167 cm)

	Normal	Observed	% predicted	Post-challenge
Spirometry				
FVC (L)	3.68	3.66	100	
FEV$_1$ (L)	3.01	2.83	94	−14
FEV$_1$/FVC (%)	82	77		
FEF$_{25-75}$ (L/s)	2.8	2.4	87	
MVV (L/min)	110	100	92	
DL$_{CO}$ (mL/min/mm Hg)	24	31	129	

Comments and Questions

This 45-year-old nurse was being treated for hypertension and complained of cough and wheezing with exertion. Physical examination was normal except for a blood pressure of 160/96 mm Hg. Her medications were not the cause of her cough. Note the negative methacholine challenge study.

1. What may be important in the data above?
2. Would you order any additional studies?

CASE 37

Answers

1. The patient is obese with a weight/height ratio of 0.72 and BMI of 42.7 kg/m². Obesity likely explains the increased D_{LCO} because the challenge was negative for asthma.
2. An exercise study was ordered and flow-volume loops were obtained. Both at rest and during exercise, as shown below, the patient breathed very near residual volume and on the expiratory limb of her maximal flow-volume curve.

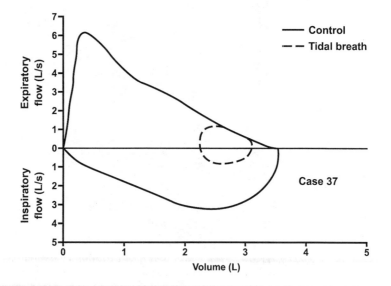

Breathing on the flow-volume curve often occurs in obese subjects and produces expiratory wheezing due to compression of the airways. Try breathing near residual volume and you likely will also wheeze. We term this "pseudoasthma," and it almost always is associated with obesity and many trips to the emergency room.

CASE 38

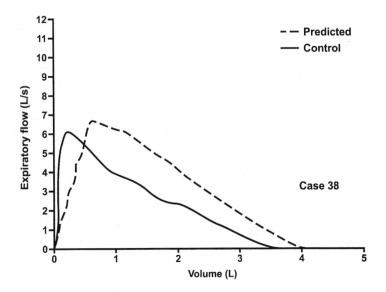

43 y   F   Wt 131 lb (59 kg)   Ht 68 in. (173 cm)

Spirometry	Normal	Observed	% predicted	Post-challenge
FVC (L)	3.93	3.81	97	2.97
FEV$_1$ (L)	3.18	2.80	88	2.18*
FEV$_1$/FVC (%)	81	73		
FEF$_{25-75}$ (L/s)	2.8	2.1	75	
MVV (L/min)	114	99	87	

Comments

The observed values are all within normal limits. However, the slope of the flow-volume curve is reduced to 1.44 L/s/L, whereas it should be 2.0 or more (see section 2F, page 13). Because of this finding and a history of episodes of bronchitis with mild dyspnea, a methacholine challenge was performed. There was a 22% decrease in the FEV$_1$ after only three breaths of methacholine (see section 5F, page 57). A reduced slope of the flow-volume curve may mean airway disease, in this case asthma (see case 16, page 175).

CASE 39

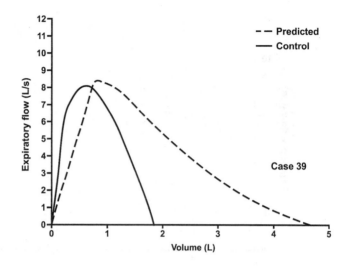

77 y   M   Wt 150 lb (68 kg)   Ht 72 in. (182 cm)

	Normal	Observed	% predicted
Spirometry			
FVC (L)	4.72	1.83*	39
FEV$_1$ (L)	3.53	1.83*	52
FEV$_1$/FVC (%)	75	99.7	
FEF$_{25-75}$ (L/s)	2.8	6.1	216
MVV (L/min)	126	93*	74
Volumes			
TLC (L)	7.16	4.75*	66
RV/TLC (%)	34	61*	179
D$_{LCO}$ (mL/min/mm Hg)	25	15*	59

Comments

There was no response to bronchodilator. Oxygen saturation was normal at rest and exercise. The shape of the flow-volume curve, reduced TLC and D$_{LCO}$, and high FEV$_1$/FVC ratio are all consistent with a parenchymal restrictive process such as fibrosis. However, the normal oximetry result is not compatible with this. The patient had congestive heart failure with bilateral pleural effusions. Basilar fibrosis was noted. Congestive heart failure can mimic pulmonary fibrosis. Contrast this case with case 18, page 179, which had a suggestion of obstruction. Thus, congestive heart failure may present with either a restrictive or an obstructive pattern.

CASE 40

Annual monitoring of change in lung function can identify persons with accelerated decline due to smoking, occupational exposures, or other causes. This person has normal lung function, which is stable over 9 years of employment. The estimated rate of decline in FEV_1 is -17 mL/y, which is normal.

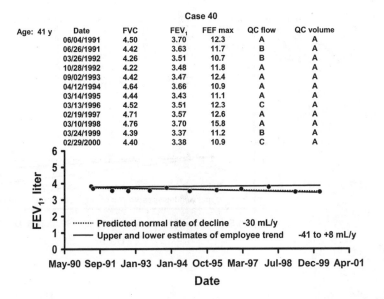

Case 40

Age: 41 y	Date	FVC	FEV₁	FEF max	QC flow	QC volume
	06/04/1991	4.50	3.70	12.3	A	A
	06/26/1991	4.42	3.63	11.7	B	A
	03/26/1992	4.26	3.51	10.7	B	A
	10/28/1992	4.22	3.48	11.8	A	A
	09/02/1993	4.42	3.47	12.4	A	A
	04/12/1994	4.64	3.66	10.9	A	A
	03/14/1995	4.44	3.43	11.1	A	A
	03/13/1996	4.52	3.51	12.3	C	A
	02/19/1997	4.71	3.57	12.6	A	A
	03/10/1998	4.76	3.70	15.8	A	A
	03/24/1999	4.39	3.37	11.2	B	A
	02/29/2000	4.40	3.38	10.9	C	A

········ Predicted normal rate of decline   -30 mL/y
─── Upper and lower estimates of employee trend   -41 to +8 mL/y

(This is an actual trend report with data from individual tests plusgrades for maneuver quality.)

CASE 41

This person, a smoker in a respiratory protection program, has had a rapid decline in lung function over 8 years. Mild obstruction has developed, and he is likely to be disabled before retirement unless appropriate preventive measures are taken. The estimated rate of decline in FEV_1 is -138 mL/y.

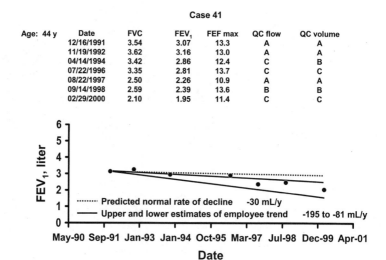

Case 41

Age: 44 y	Date	FVC	FEV$_1$	FEF max	QC flow	QC volume
	12/16/1991	3.54	3.07	13.3	A	A
	11/19/1992	3.62	3.16	13.0	A	A
	04/14/1994	3.42	2.86	12.4	C	B
	07/22/1996	3.35	2.81	13.7	C	C
	08/22/1997	2.50	2.26	10.9	A	A
	09/14/1998	2.59	2.39	13.6	B	B
	02/29/2000	2.10	1.95	11.4	C	C

Predicted normal rate of decline   -30 mL/y
Upper and lower estimates of employee trend   -195 to -81 mL/y

CASE 42

More frequent monitoring may be needed for persons with labile lung function, such as those with asthma, and for persons with lung injury or lung transplantation. This trend shows gradual improvement in lung function of an employee of a chemical plant who was exposed to chlorine in an industrial accident. Lung function improved rapidly during the first month after his injury, then slowly during the following 5 years.

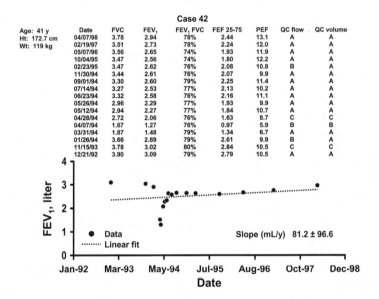

Case 42

Age: 41 y	Date	FVC	FEV₁	FEV/FVC	FEF 25-75	PEF	QC flow	QC volume
Ht: 172.7 cm	04/07/98	3.78	2.94	78%	2.44	13.1	A	A
Wt: 119 kg	02/19/97	3.51	2.73	78%	2.24	12.0	A	A
	05/07/96	3.56	2.65	74%	1.93	11.9	A	A
	10/04/95	3.47	2.56	74%	1.80	12.2	A	A
	02/23/95	3.47	2.62	76%	2.08	10.8	B	A
	11/30/94	3.44	2.61	76%	2.07	9.9	A	A
	09/01/94	3.30	2.60	79%	2.25	11.4	A	A
	07/14/94	3.27	2.53	77%	2.13	10.2	A	A
	06/23/94	3.32	2.58	76%	2.16	11.1	A	A
	05/26/94	2.96	2.29	77%	1.93	9.9	A	A
	05/12/94	2.94	2.27	77%	1.84	10.7	A	A
	04/28/94	2.72	2.06	76%	1.63	8.7	C	C
	04/07/94	1.67	1.27	76%	0.97	5.9	B	B
	03/31/94	1.87	1.48	79%	1.34	6.7	A	A
	01/26/94	3.66	2.89	79%	2.61	9.9	B	A
	11/15/93	3.78	3.02	80%	2.84	10.5	C	C
	12/21/92	3.90	3.09	79%	2.79	10.5	A	A

CASE 43

This trend from a patient who had lung transplantation shows gradual improvement over 2 months, then an episode of rejection, which was treated successfully 7 months after transplantation. Values indicated by an "X" were deleted from analysis because they were "outliers" caused by a wet flow element.

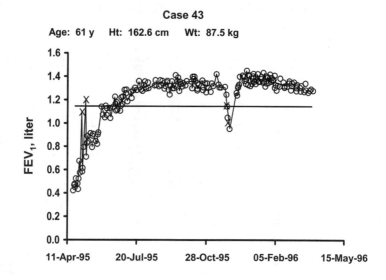

Case 43

Age: 61 y   Ht: 162.6 cm   Wt: 87.5 kg

CASE 44

This trend shows the progressive decline in function of a patient with obliterative bronchiolitis after lung transplantation.

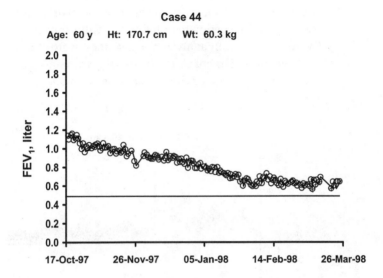

CASE 45

This trend is highly variable with frequent "spikes" showing arti-
factual increases in FEV_1. These were due to the patient's use of
a wet spirometer flow sensor. The moisture increases the flow resistance of the element, giving an increase in driving pressure and
causing an overestimate of his FEV_1. Values indicated by an "X"
were deleted from analysis because they were "outliers" caused
by a wet flow element. After the patient was reinstructed in proper
care of the spirometer, the artifact was eliminated.

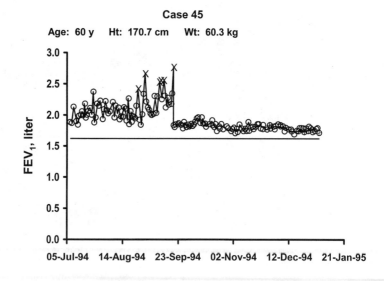

Case 45

Age: 60 y   Ht: 170.7 cm   Wt: 60.3 kg

TYPES OF CASES

Appendix

Normal values are used in this text to construct predicted normal flow-volume curves.

The flow-volume curves are predicted on the basis of four predicted flow points and the predicted forced expiratory vital capacity (FVC). The value for peak expiratory flow (PEF) is plotted after 12.5% of the predicted FVC has been exhaled and connected to the zero flow-zero exhaled volume point by a straight line. Next, predicted flows after 25, 50, and 75% of the predicted FVC have been exhaled are plotted at their appropriate volumes. The PEF, FEF_{25}, FEF_{50}, and FEF_{75} are connected by straight lines. The FEF_{75} is also connected to the volume point at 100% of the predicted FVC at which flow is zero.

The equations listed on the following page are used to predict the mean values of the various flows and of the FVC. Age (A) is in years, and standing height (H) is in centimeters or meters (H/100).

TABLE A-1. Equations for predicting FVC and various flows

	Age (y)	Male	Age (y)	Female
FVC	5–11	$4.4 \times 10^{-6} \times H^{2.67}$	5–10	$3.3 \times 10^{-6} \times H^{2.72}$
	12–19	$0.0590 \times H + 0.0739$ $\times A - 6.89$	11–19	$0.0416 \times H + 0.0699$ $\times A - 4.45$
	20+	$0.0774 \times H - 0.0212$ $\times A - 7.75$	20+	$0.0414 \times H - 0.0232$ $\times A - 2.198$
PEF	5–11	$2.12 \times (H/100)^{2.79}$	5–10	$2.36 \times (H/100)^{2.37}$
	12–19	$0.078 \times H + 0.166$ $\times A - 8.06$	11–19	$0.049 \times H + 0.157$ $\times A - 3.92$
	20+	$0.094 \times H - 0.035$ $\times A - 5.99$	20+	$0.049 \times H - 0.025$ $\times A - 0.74$
FEF_{25}	5–11	$0.078 \times H - 6.82$	5–10	$0.064 \times H - 5.19$
	12–19	$0.070 \times H + 0.147$ $\times A - 7.05$	11–19	$0.044 \times H + 0.144$ $\times A - 3.37$
	20+	$0.088 \times H - 0.035$ $\times A - 5.62$	20+	$0.043 \times H - 0.025$ $\times A - 0.13$
FEF_{50}	5–11	$0.05 \times H - 4.58$	5–10	$0.045 \times H - 3.37$
	12–19	$0.0543 \times H + 0.1150$ $\times A - 6.39$	11–19	$0.0288 \times H + 0.1111$ $\times A - 2.30$
	20+	$0.0684 \times H - 0.0366$ $\times A - 5.54$	20–69	$0.0321 \times H - 0.0240$ $\times A - 0.44$
			70+	$0.0118 \times H - 0.0755$ $\times A + 6.24$
FEF_{75}	5–11	$0.028 \times H - 2.31$	5–10	$0.025 \times H - 1.86$
	12–19	$0.0397 \times H - 0.0057$ $\times A - 4.24$	11–19	$0.0243 \times H + 0.2923$ $\times A - 0.0075 \times A^2 - 4.4$
	20+	$0.0310 \times H - 0.0230$ $\times A - 2.48$	20–69	$0.0174 \times H - 0.0254$ $\times A - 0.18$
			70+	$-0.0172 \times A + 1.89$

Subject Index

Page numbers followed by f *indicate a figure;* t *following a page number indicates tabular material*